Good Foods, Bad Foods

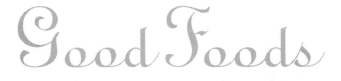

Bad Foods

Suzanne Havala, M.S., R.D.

CHRONIMED PUBLISHING

Library of Congress Cataloging-in-Publication Data

Havala, Suzanne

Good foods, bad foods: what's left to eat? / Suzanne Havala

p.   cm.

ISBN 1-56561-171-3: $19.95

Acquiring Editor: Jeff Braun
Editor: Alice Kelly
Cover Design: Max Media
Text Design & Production: David Enyeart
Art/Production Manager: Claire Lewis

Printed in the United States

Published by
CHRONIMED PUBLISHING
P.O. Box 59032
Minneapolis, MN 55459-0032

10   9   8   7   6   5   4   3   2   1

Acknowledgments vii

About the Author ix

Part One: Cutting Through the Confusion

1. Talking Politics 3

2. They Say, "Eat a Variety of Foods" 25

3. They Say, "Balance Your Food with Physical Activity" 41

4. They Say, "Choose a Diet with Plenty of Grains, Vegetables, and Fruits"... 51

5. They Say, "Choose a Diet Low in Fat, Saturated Fat, and Cholesterol" 61

6. They Say, "Choose a Diet Moderate in Sugar, Salt, and Sodium" 71

7. Summary: The Simple Truth 81

Part Two: Getting from Here to There

8. The Optimal Diet is Outside Our Culture 89

9. Making the Change At Home 93

10. Eating Out.. 109

11. The Social Side 123

12. Traveling Light 131

13. How to Get Support 145

14. A Simple Meal-Planning Guide 153

15. Menus Made Easy.. 163

16. Recipe Modifications 173

Recommended Dietary Allowances and Dietary Reference Intakes 185

Index 191

To my parents

Acknowledgments

One of the greatest joys of writing a book of this nature is the opportunity to interact with so many friends and colleagues and to make some valued new acquaintances along the way, as well. Indeed, rather than a book written in isolation, this book is the result of the contributions of many individuals who went out of their way to lend me support, encouragement, advice, technical expertise, and their own unique points of view.

Chief among those is my friend and literary agent, Patti Breitman, whose unflagging enthusiasm, interest, and words of wisdom helped to support and guide this project. I have the greatest admiration and respect for my editor at Chronimed Publishing, Jeff Braun, with whom I was delighted to have had the opportunity to work on a second book. It is a privilege to have the opportunity to work with such a fine team as the staff at Chronimed. In particular, I would like to thank David Enyeart and Alice Kelly.

I owe a debt of gratitude to my friends and colleagues who took the time from their own busy lives to read and discuss my manuscript and offer thoughtful comments. Deepest thanks to Kathleen Babich, R.N., B.S.N.; T. Colin Campbell, Ph.D. (Cornell University, Ithaca, N.Y.); Mary Clifford, R.D.; Winston Craig, Ph.D., R.D. (Andrews University, Berrien Springs, Mich.); Michael Jacobson, Ph.D. (Center for Science in the Public Interest, Washington, D.C.); Reed Mangels, Ph.D., R.D., (The Vegetarian Resource Group, Baltimore, Md.); Mark Messina, Ph.D. and Virginia Messina, M.P.H., R.D. (Nutrition Matters, Inc., Port Townsend, Wash.); Charles Stahler (The Vegetarian Resource Group, Baltimore, Md.); and Robert C. Wesley Jr., M.D. (University of Nevada School of Medicine, Las Vegas, Nevada).

Many thanks to the chefs and restaurant owners who so generously and enthusiastically shared their insights and advice about eating out: Jody Adams (Chef, Rialto, Cambridge, Mass.); Robert Del Grande (Chef/Partner, Cafe Annie, Houston, Texas); Mark Dowling (Chef/Instructor, The Disney Institute, Orlando, Fla.); Susan Feniger and Mary Sue Milliken (Owners, Border Grill, Santa Monica, Calif.); David Garrido (Executive Chef, Jeffrey's, Austin, Texas); Theresa Girault (Owner, Carpe Diem, Charlotte, N.C.), Tom Maier (President, Agri-Culinary Enterprises, and Chef, Cavanaugh's, Kalispell, Mont.); Peter Merriman (Owner, Merriman's Restaurant, Waimea, Hawaii); Caprial Pence (Owner, Caprial's, Portland, Ore.); Odessa Piper (Executive Chef and Proprietor, L'Etoile, Madison, Wisc.), Michael Romano (Executive Chef/Partner, Union Square Cafe, New York, N.Y.); Burniece Rott (Executive Chef, Nature's Fresh Northwest, Portland, Ore.); Stewart Scruggs (Executive Chef, Zoot, Austin, Texas); Gary Sloss (Executive Chef, The Forest Country Club, Ft. Myers, Fla.); Ana Sortun (Chef, Casablanca, Cambridge, Mass.); Elizabeth Terry (Owner, Elizabeth on 37th, Savannah, Ga.); and Lynn Walters (Chef and Owner, Natural Cafe, Santa Fe, N.M.).

I am also grateful for the ongoing support of my friends and colleagues in Vegetarian Nutrition, a dietetic practice group of the American Dietetic Association, as well as the staff and volunteers of The Vegetarian Resource Group.

Finally, I am very fortunate to have a close circle of family and friends who are an ever-present source of love, encouragement, support, and humor. Foremost among those are my parents, Milt and Kay Babich, whose dedication and support have gone well beyond the call of duty. My sisters and brother, Sandra Babich (and Sarah and Scott); Julie Covington and Wayne, her new husband; and David Babich form the hub of my immediate family, with spokes that include dear cousins, other extended family, and friends that are family to me. These relationships are among my greatest sources of joy.

A great many individuals have inspired and supported me in my work, and this list only begins to acknowledge those to whom I am indebted. I am grateful to and appreciate one and all.

About the Author

---◇---

Suzanne Havala, M.S., R.D., L.D.N., F.A.D.A., is a licensed, registered dietitian and professional nutrition consultant. In addition to working with food companies, nonprofit groups, and other organizations, she writes books and articles, appears on radio and television, and lectures to professionals and the general public. Among her special areas of interest are health promotion, food trends, and vegetarian diets.

She was the primary author of the American Dietetic Association's 1988 and 1993 position papers on vegetarian diets, and she is a founding member and former chairperson of the ADA's Vegetarian Nutrition Dietetic Practice Group. She is a nutrition adviser for the national, nonprofit Vegetarian Resource Group, and she serves on the editorial advisory board of *Vegetarian Times* magazine.

She is a past member of the American Dietetic Association's State Media Representative/Ambassador Program. She is a regular contributor to *Vegetarian Journal*, and she has written for *Vegetarian Times*, *Environmental Nutrition Newsletter*, and other magazines and newsletters. She is frequently quoted in national magazines and newspapers, such as *The New York Times*, *Parade*, *Shape*, *Runner's World*, *New Woman*, YM, *Omni*, *Sassy*, *Harper's Bazaar*, and many others, and has appeared on Good Morning America, the Susan Powter Show, and Weekend Today in New York.

Ms. Havala is the author of *The Vegetarian Food Guide and Nutrition Counter* (Berkley Publishing, 1997); the American Dietetic Association's guide to vegetarian diets, *Being Vegetarian* (Chronimed, 1996); *Shopping for Health*: A *Nutritionist's Aisle-by-Aisle Guide to Smart, Low-Fat Choices at the Supermarket* (HarperPerennial, 1996); and *Simple, Lowfat & Vegetarian* (The Vegetarian Resource Group, 1994). She is the co-creator of the "Shopping for Health" video series (Family Experiences Productions Inc., 1997).

Ms. Havala is certified as a charter Fellow of the American Dietetic Association, a status granted to only 1% of the nearly 70,000 members of the ADA. She holds a bachelor of science degree with honor in dietetics from Michigan State University and a master of science degree in human nutrition from Winthrop University, Rock Hill, S.C. Currently, she is based in Chapel Hill, N.C., where she is a doctoral student majoring in health policy and administration in the School of Public Health at the University of North Carolina.

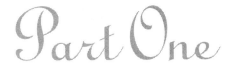

Part One

Cutting Through the Confusion

Chapter One

Talking Politics

"I've read so much about the dangers of eating that I've decided to give up reading."

Sound familiar? You may think it's a joke. But to millions of people who are trying to lose weight, lower their cholesterol levels, and stay well, it's no laughing matter. They're confused, and it's no wonder.

The connection between diet and health is well established. Eat right, and you stand a good chance of preventing or delaying the onset of coronary artery disease, diabetes, high blood pressure, some types of cancer, obesity, and other diseases and conditions. If you already have a problem, changing your diet may help treat it. Losing weight and boosting fiber intake, for example, can help diabetics control their blood sugar levels and reduce or eliminate their need for insulin injections or other medications. Research has shown that dietary changes can help to reverse even severe coronary artery disease, causing regression of plaque buildup in the arteries.

"Sounds great," you say. "How do I begin?"

That's the catch. That's where the confusion comes in. For all the talk about diet and health, there is precious little direct advice about what to eat. You have a better chance of winning the lottery than you have of hitting on clear and accurate advice about what to eat and how to make the changes.

Think about it. You read in the paper one day that beta carotene can prevent heart disease, so you eat more carrots. A year later, you read that another study has linked beta carotene with cancer. Nutritionists say you should eat less fat and cholesterol. But they also say "there are no good foods or bad foods" and that anything can fit into a balanced diet. They say, "Eat more fiber, but don't eat too much."

Dietary messages are conflicting and as clear as mud. No, there's no need to stop reading or eating, but there is a desperate need to expose and clarify the truths that are buried deep within the dietary recommendations that we read and hear about in the media and from health professionals.

Why is Everything So Confusing?

You pay diligent attention to food and nutrition stories in the news, and you take to heart dietary recommendations made by reputable sources. You pick up books on diet and health and do your best to educate yourself on the issues. You are a conscientious consumer, and you want to take responsibility for your own health.

So why is it so hard to figure out what to eat for dinner tonight?

If you find yourself in this state of perplexity, you're not stupid, and you're not alone. You're caught up in the never-ending cycle of nutrition doublespeak, lost in the murky waters of an area of science—human nutrition—that is still in its infancy. Above all, you're a victim of the politics of your plate.

It should be noted at the outset that some of the confusion people feel concerning dietary recommendations stems from the simple fact that science as we know it is always changing. Nothing in nutrition is carved in stone, and what we know today will, no doubt, be improved by future research.

When I was in college in the late 1970s and early 1980s, physicians considered cholesterol levels of up to 300 milligrams per deciliter to be normal. Today, your doctor would have a heart attack if your cholesterol level were that high. Coronary care units routinely served patients bacon and eggs for breakfast, and in class, I learned about the Pritikin diet and vegetarianism in the unit on fad diets. How times have changed.

The point is, we are only beginning to understand the complexities of human nutrition. Become comfortable with the fact that recommendations will change over time. The key is not to react too quickly when the media brings attention to the findings of a single research study. University researchers (and special interest groups that sponsor some of the research) have become very media savvy in recent years and frequently seek press attention for their research findings. It's not your imagination; there's a new study mentioned in the news almost every day.

Generally, it's not until research findings are replicated by other researchers, and there is a big enough body of research upon which to base consensus, that changes in dietary recommendations are warranted. (There might be exceptions. In the case of a food safety issue—let's say, a particular food was found to be contaminated with a dangerous chemical—it might be wise to stop eating that food right away, instead of waiting for several studies to confirm the presence of the contaminant.) The best approach is to keep abreast of the news but to maintain a "big picture" mentality.

Is oat bran being touted for its cholesterol-lowering potential? Here's an example of how I would handle nutrition news. What do the researchers think it is about oat bran that causes this cholesterol-lowering effect? It's the soluble fiber? Okay. Which other foods are high in soluble fiber? Beans, fruits, and vegetables. Since I know that these foods are good for me anyway, I'd just make an extra effort to include plenty of all of them in my diet. That's the big-picture approach. Makes more sense than eating bushels of oat bran. There are no "magic bullet" foods or nutrients. But sometimes research findings like this one are clues that can validate or challenge broader dietary recommendations.

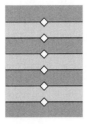

Pol.i.tics

3 a : political affairs or business; specif: competition between competing interest groups or individuals for power and leadership in a government or other group ... c : political activities characterized by artful and often dishonest practices

—*Webster's New Collegiate Dictionary*

The Politics of Your Plate

Then, of course, there is the politics. It never really bothered anybody, say, back in the 1940s and 1950s, when the National Dairy Council produced its "Guide to Good Eating," which was used by elementary schools everywhere for decades to teach the fundamentals of nutrition. Based on the Basic Four Food Groups dietary model, it depicted dairy products—milk, cheese, ice cream—as one of the four cornerstones of a "balanced" diet. Never mind that the concept was the ultimate marketing tool for the dairy industry. The focus then was on preventing dietary deficiencies, and the nutritional merits of dairy products were emphasized exclusively. Recognition of and concerns about excesses in the American diet—too much fat, cholesterol, and protein—were many years away. Besides, milk was as American as apple pie. Who could find fault with that?

Fast forward to 1980, the year that the U.S. Departments of Agriculture (USDA) and Health and Human Services (HHS) jointly published the first Dietary Guidelines for Americans. Targeting every person over the age of two years, the Dietary Guidelines give advice about food choices that promote health and lessen the risk for disease. Revisions of the report were published in 1985, 1990, and 1995.

The Dietary Guidelines are the cornerstone of federal nutrition policy. As of 1990, legislation requires that the report be published every five years by the secretaries of USDA and HHS. The information is directed to the general public, must be based on the preponderance of scientific and medical knowledge current at the time of publication, and is to be promoted by USDA, HHS, and other federal agencies.

So the USDA is in the business of giving dietary advice to the American public. That's a sideline, however. The USDA's primary reason for being is to support American agriculture. The biggest players—and the most powerful, given their financial clout—are the meat and dairy industries. A conflict of interest? You bet. Does it influence what the Dietary Guidelines say? Absolutely.

Insiders will tell you about the impact this conflict has had on U.S. nutrition policy over the years. For instance, in 1977, when Sen. George McGovern's Senate Select Committee on Nutrition made recommendations for the first set of Dietary Guidelines, the committee suggested, among other things, that the guidelines should clearly state that people should cut down on high-cholesterol foods and should further note that meat is high in cholesterol. Buckling under pressure from representatives from the meat industry, however, the reference to meat was stricken from the final report. Instead, the report stated that people should "avoid too much fat, saturated fat, and cholesterol," and left it at that.

It has long been in industry's interest to support dietary guidelines that are relatively vague and "open to interpretation." The meat, dairy, and egg industries, in particular, would stand to lose if dietary guidelines were more specific and people began eating fewer of their products. It's that very ambiguity, however, that vexes the public and annoys consumer advocates. Without clear-cut guidelines that name names and give specific recommendations that get to the nitty-gritty of what people should eat, everyone is left standing at square one saying, "I've read the guidelines, and that's all well and good, but *what do I eat for dinner tonight?*"

After the publication of the 1995 revision of the Dietary Guidelines, reporter Sally Squires noted in the January 3, 1996, issue of *The Washington Post* that "moderation in all things" appears to be the basic message of the government's dietary guidelines. She wrote, "Critics complained that the new recommendations don't go far enough," and quoted Michael Jacobson, executive director of the Center for Science in the Public Interest, who stated, "The dietary guidelines should be telling the public what is the best possible diet. These guidelines don't."

The 1995 Dietary Guidelines Advisory Committee acknowledged that consumers have not been successful overall in translating the Dietary Guidelines into lifestyle changes and recommended that future revisions of the Dietary Guidelines take this problem into consideration. To investigate the issue further, the USDA and HHS sponsored consumer-based research in the spring of 1995. The findings: Consumers want straightforward advice with specific directions. Consumers do not have the time, energy, or inclination to learn nutrition science before they can begin to eat a healthful diet. No surprise here.

In the meantime, an alliance of food industry and health organizations, in liaison with the federal government, was formed in 1996 to develop materials that will help consumers translate the Dietary Guidelines and put them into practice. Called the Dietary Guidelines Alliance, the group includes, along with the USDA and HHS, the American Dietetic Association, the Food Marketing Institute, the International Food Information Council, the National Dairy Council, the National Food Processors Association, the National Cattlemen's Beef Association, the Produce Marketing Association, the Sugar Association, the Wheat Foods Council, and the National Pork Producers Council.

Once again, that's the politics of your plate.

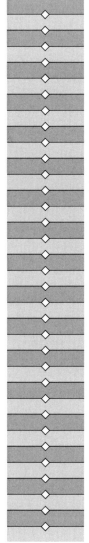

what's left to eat?

From a September 17, 1996, *New York Times* article titled "Society Issues a Tough New Warning on Diet" (in reference to new dietary guidelines issued by the American Cancer Society):

The society made four main recommendations yesterday, which appear to be similar to current dietary advice that comes from the Government ...

In the details, however, the guidelines are very different from those provided by the government, and some health experts attribute that difference to the pressures that are brought to bear on the government by groups that could be hurt financially. Dr. Marion Nestle, chairman of the advisory committee that developed the guidelines for the society and chairman of the department of nutrition and food studies at New York University, said the advice came from a group that had no other agenda than "helping people prevent, treat, and cure cancer."

Dr. Meir Stampfer, a professor of epidemiology and nutrition at the Harvard School of Public Health, said the cancer society, unlike the federal government, "is in a position to make guidelines based more strictly on science." The government, said Dr. Stampfer, who was not a member of the panel, "is subject to economic pressure as well as scientific pressure."

The government recommends eating lean meat and limiting consumption of high-fat meats like sausage and salami. The society recommends curtailing all red meat, not just high-fat meat. It links consumption of red meat to colon and prostate cancer.

"It is inappropriate to indict meat," said Dr. Janet William, the vice president of scientific and technical affairs for the American Meat Institute, a trade group. "The document is not consistent with U.S. Dietary Guidelines."

The Art of Nutrition Doublespeak, or
What They Say Isn't What They Mean

In the realm of nutrition politics, things get curiouser and curiouser. Why is it, for instance, that when nutritionists give dietary advice, it can never really be translated into concrete actions? You just can't nail it down. "The keys to a healthful eating style are balance, variety, and moderation. There are no good or bad foods, only good or bad diets." What on Earth does it mean? Should I eat the chili dog or not?

Mainstream nutritionists are trained to understand diet from an American perspective, with an inherent philosophy that "you start from where people are at, and you don't try to change them." For instance, if someone is a vegetarian, you work with that and don't try to convince them to eat meat. And vice versa. We dietitians all learned this basic value in school.

Where the vast majority of Americans are "at", of course, is a traditional American diet, the ol' balanced diet concept. A meal revolves around a piece of meat, then we add the starch, a couple of vegetables, and a piece of fruit for dessert (apple pie counts). The assumption at the root of dietary recommendations in the U.S., as well as in the system that educates American nutritionists, is that our American model is not going to change. This is our tradition, and this is the way we like it.

This philosophy extends to the establishment of nutrient standards, as well. A good example is the Recommended Dietary Allowance (RDA) for calcium. (RDAs are the levels of intake of essential nutrients that the Food and Nutrition Board judges to be adequate to meet the known nutrient needs of practically all healthy persons.) Americans consume excessive amounts of protein, which, along with excessive intakes of sodium, causes an increased loss of calcium through the urine. Rather than counseling people to reduce their protein intake (which would conflict with the traditional American eating pattern), the committee jacked up the recommended level of calcium intake enough (it hoped) to compensate for the calcium losses.

The RDA for calcium is set so high that it is essentially impossible to meet unless one takes a calcium supplement or consumes foods that are superconcentrated in calcium, such as cow's milk. If one consumes the recommended number of servings of dairy products every day, fat, cholesterol, and protein intakes usually increase and fiber intake decreases, since dairy products are devoid of fiber. The end result, then, is at odds with current recommendations to eat less fat and cholesterol and more fiber. Problems are perpetuated, but the traditional eating pattern is preserved.

And it gets even murkier. The American nutrition establishment has a long history of partnership with the food industry. For decades, industry has provided substantial funding for everything from nutrition research and nutrition education programs to professional conferences and other activities. Almost every dietitian in the country has directly benefited from industry dollars. On the local level, industry often pays for the printing of dietetic association newsletters, donates money or supplies for meetings, and pays for an occasional lunch or dinner out. On the national level, industry donates big money to support professional association operations.

The American Dietetic Association (ADA) is one of several professional organizations that has benefited from and grown to depend on financial support from industry. The ADA is the largest group of nutrition professionals in the world, with more than 70,000 members. In addition to the parent organization, the ADA has state and local dietetic association affiliates. Most college and university nutrition programs strongly encourage their students to join the ADA, and some employers consider membership in the ADA to be a condition of employment.

In the January 1996 issue of the ADA *Courier*, a publication of the American Dietetic Association mailed monthly to members, then-President Doris Derelian wrote, "As many of you know, The American Dietetic Association's nutrition education philosophies have been the subject of some public scrutiny of late. In a recent newspaper article, for example, it was suggested that because ADA receives some financial support from food companies, our educational messages for the public might be negatively influenced."

It isn't difficult to understand how one could come to the conclusion that financial dependence might color the messages that a group like the ADA gives the public. The ADA is, first and foremost, a membership organization. It exists to serve its members and promote the profession of dietetics. Industry money has enabled the organization to fund initiatives that would never have been possible otherwise.

In the April 1996 issue of the ADA *Courier*, for instance, a column titled, "Industry partners support Consumer Nutrition Hot Line," noted that the "ADA Foundation and the National Center for Nutrition and Dietetics [the NCND is the ADA's public education initiative] acknowledges the following

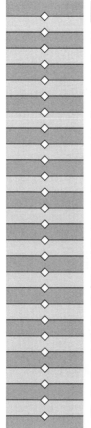

what's left to eat?

Industry Groups Have an "In" on Educating the Public

Should professionals permit industry groups to promote their products via the professionals' organizations, such as the American Dietetic Association? Does money given to professional groups by industry to promote specific food products influence the nutrition messages that the public receives from those groups?

In the August 1996 issue of the *ADA Courier,* the American Dietetic Association thanks its industry partners for supporting the ADA's Consumer Nutrition Hot Line and notes that the July 1996 recorded message for consumers—"Healthy Meals Sizzle with Flavor When Cooked on the Grill"—was sponsored by the National Pork Producers Council.

In the same issue, the *Courier* notes, "The National Dairy Council joins Kellogg in ADA's Child Nutrition Health Campaign with a grant to provide funding for hot line messages, nutrition fact sheets, and their placement in the Journal of the American Dietetic Association, along with support for expert panel and annual meeting activities. The National Dairy Council will also support a 30-second TV public service announcement that will tell children about the importance of breakfast and performance. This will be augmented by an advertorial scheduled to appear in a high-circulation magazine later this year."

industry partners for their support of the Consumer Nutrition Hot Line through recorded messages and nutrition fact sheets ..."

Industry groups listed were Best Foods Inc., makers of Mazola — "The ABCs of Fats, Oils, and Cholesterol" (Spanish); The Coca-Cola Company and the National Osteoporosis Foundation — "Choose Calcium-rich Foods for Strong Bones"; and The National Cattlemen's Beef Association — "The Lean 'n Easy Way to Enjoy Meat."

Cola drinks are high in phosphates, which increase the loss of calcium from bone. Why would Coca-Cola want to fund a consumer message on osteoporosis? All of the industry groups involved in these messages produce products that people would be better off avoiding. Added fats and oils, sugary soft drinks that are high in phosphates, and meat are all food items that Americans consume in excess and that are implicated by research, in the amounts generally consumed, to be detrimental to our health. Hmmmm.

Let's go back to the column from the January 1996 issue of the ADA *Courier*—the column focusing on the nutrition education philosophy of the ADA. In response to accusations that the ADA's educational messages to the public might be influenced by its industry relationships, then-President Doris Derelian continues:

"This is simply not true. ADA's nutrition education philosophies are based on sound science. All of our public education efforts are based on the following principles:

- There are no good or bad foods, only good or bad diets.
- The keys to a healthful eating style are balance, variety, and moderation.
- Messages should focus on the total diet, not individual foods.
- A positive approach to eating should be emphasized.
- Increased physical activity is beneficial.

"One question often raised is why ADA says there are no good or bad foods. Well, the Recommended Dietary Allowances (RDAs) and 1995 Dietary Guidelines for Americans are, according to the guidelines, based on 'diets consumed over several days and not [on] single meals or foods.'"

The column continues:

"Based on that principle, it's clear that any food can fit into a healthful eating style…. the charge of the dietetics professional—as the food and nutrition expert—is not to insist that people give up their favorite foods… —because all foods contribute some essential nutrients.

"As an organization with limited resources, we are indeed fortunate, on occasion, to find like-minded partners in the corporate world willing to fund our efforts and, in the process, help us educate millions more consumers than we could reach on the strength of our own resources.

"The bottom line: ADA enters into partnerships exclusively with companies that support our philosophies. In this way, we continue to ensure the integrity of all our education efforts."

As far as the consumer is concerned, however, the real bottom line is anything goes. That is the message conveyed by statements such as "There are no good foods or bad foods" and "All foods contribute some essential nutrients."

Do you remember the naturalist Euell Gibbons of *Stalking the Wild Asparagus* fame? I have memories of him in television commercials for breakfast cereal, strolling through a meadow, stopping next to a pine tree and eating a piece of the bark. Mmmm. Fiber.

Sure, pine bark contains some essential nutrients, but that doesn't mean I'd recommend that you eat it. By not taking a stand and stating that some foods are better than others, by not citing specifics and being more direct, nutrition education messages are clouded and obscure. Have you ever listened to a politician speak for a great length of time, only to realize later that he or she said nothing of substance? No particular point was made, but no one was offended, either.

In the case of your diet, many American nutritionists have mastered the art of nutrition doublespeak. By avoiding specifics, nobody steps on anybody else's toes. You say you've been reading and listening to dietary advice and trying your darnedest to do it right, but you still can't figure out what to make for dinner tonight? It's not you. It's them. They've been talking in circles, speaking without actually making a point.

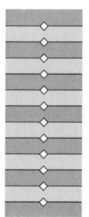

What's left to eat?

Do you worry that the foods you love—like steak, eggs and milkshakes—are unhealthful or, worse, unsafe? "There's no such thing as a 'bad' food or a food that causes disease," says Kristine Clark, the director of sports nutrition at Penn State University and nutritionist for the U.S. women's Olympic soccer and field hockey teams. Clark raised some eyebrows when she told the athletes that red meat and eggs are part of a healthy diet. "All foods are good," she says. "Only the amounts you eat could be bad."

—From an article in the November 17, 1996 issue
of *Parade* magazine, titled "Don't Fear Your Food"

No Good Foods, No Bad Foods

When nutritionists say there are "no good or bad foods, only good or bad diets," they often add the caveat that one cannot assign moral qualities to foods. Okay, so the salami isn't guilty of clogging your arteries. It was you who put it on your menu. As opponents of gun control will tell you, the hand that pulls the trigger is the guilty party, not the gun itself.

I look at the issue a little differently. Personally, when I say that a food is "good" or "bad," I am referring to the food's relative value in terms of health. A "good" food is one that promotes health. A "bad" food is one that is comparatively worse for you. A bad food is a food that, eaten in sufficient quantities, either contributes to nutritional excesses or displaces more valuable foods from the diet.

As Marian Burros, food writer for *The New York Times*, once opined, "Regarding good foods/bad foods: There are some foods that are better than others. If you don't want to use the term 'bad foods,' then there are foods and there are good foods. The good foods you can eat anytime and the foods you can eat occasionally."

Over the many years that I have been counseling people on diet and nutrition, one need has always risen above all others. That is, people want specific advice about what they should and should not eat, preferably with the emphasis on the good choices. They want to know what they can have for dinner tonight. They want concrete examples of good foods to order at restaurants, and they want lists of good snack ideas.

One of the ADA's "key messages" for National Nutrition Month 1996 was, "Any food in today's diverse marketplace fits in a healthful eating style." The theme for 1997 was "All foods can fit."

Sure. A chocolate chip cookie can be worked in each day if the rest of the diet is up to snuff. Dietary recommendations don't have to be strictly black or white, eat this and don't eat that. There is some gray area, some room for play and for individualizing the diet.

But most Americans are light years away from meeting current dietary recommendations. There are certainly some very specific tips that could be given that would be relevant to the majority. That means identifying some foods as being better choices than others. If the vague statements that are now the norm are not backed up strongly with specific recommendations that name names and define terms, then people will not be able to make the kinds of dietary changes that they need to make in order to see significant health benefits.

An article by Marian Burros in the November 15, 1995 issue of *The New York Times* explored the sticky issue of health professional associations accepting industry monies and in-kind services. She quoted Joan Gussow, Ph.D., a former head of the nutrition education program at Columbia University's Teachers College, who stated that the American Dietetic Association's dependence on industry money meant that "they never criticize the food industry." The ADA won't finger any particular food as being bad, unhealthful, or a poor choice. Even candy bars and soft drinks have a place, according to the ADA. "Actually, we could put our name on any McDonald's meal," said Dr. Doris Derelian, who was the current president of the American Dietetic Association.

In the same article, Dr. Gussow also stated, "If health professionals are led to agree that there are no 'good' or 'bad,' 'healthy' or 'unhealthy' foods, then we can't object to any food product that's put on the market, however wasteful or useless it may be."

She added, "The food critics of the '60s and '70s have been silenced, which is, of course, the point. The food industry prefers it that way."

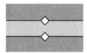 **"In this country, we're dying of moderation."**
—Robert Pritikin, director of the Pritikin Longevity Centers

"Variety, Balance, and Moderation Are the Keys"

Another of the ADA's key messages for National Nutrition Month 1996 was, "An eating style with food variety as well as balance and moderation maximizes lifelong fitness." What does this mean?

The statement that there are no good or bad foods is often followed by the equally vague concept that variety, balance, and moderation are the keys to a healthful diet. What does this mean to a person for whom breakfast is a sausage-egg-and-cheese biscuit, lunch is a Big Mac and a Coke, and dinner consists of a "balanced" meal of a pork chop, mashed potatoes with gravy, iceberg lettuce salad with bleu cheese dressing, and a glass of milk? Does the salad balance the pork chop? Is moderation having a small Coke instead of a large? Does variety mean having chicken for dinner one night and beef the next?

The reality is that these terms mean little to anyone. We are a culture with such extremes in diet that a little tweaking here and there does not result in changes substantial enough to promote significant health benefits.

Politics enters into the frequent use of these terms as well. Take the term "moderation."

Bonnie Liebman, Director of Nutrition for the Center for Science in the Public Interest, has said, "I never use the term because it's too vague, and the food industry uses it as a smoke-screen to make people think whatever they're eating is okay."

Moderation. It seems so reasonable. So sane. It's a pacifier, especially when someone has the audacity to suggest that there might be something wrong with a steak at Morton's.

It bears repeating: If we were at the point of fine-tuning our diets, the term "moderation" might be relevant. But given the starting point for most people in our culture—such extremes in diet composition—the term loses its meaning.

Then there are "variety" and "balance." Increasingly, these words come into play when discussions about dietary recommendations get close to "naming names" and citing specific advice about food choices.

Why? Because the science is becoming difficult to ignore, and as research overwhelmingly points to the need for Americans to move to a more plant-based diet, this creates serious conflict. A move to a plant-based diet is a threat to the American way. Not only do we have an animal-based agricultural system, with many who stand to lose if meat and dairy products are relegated to the side of the plate or are pushed off all together, but we have a tradition of a certain way of eating.

Traditions are hard to shake. Ask anyone who has tried to overhaul his or her diet how difficult it is to change. Try eating out at a restaurant, inviting guests over for dinner, or being the guest in someone's else's home. Try finding a replacement for Aunt Dee's cream cheese brownies or simply letting go of the idea that a meal has to center around a piece of meat.

Changing lifelong habits and replacing old traditions with new ones is tough. It's uncomfortable. No wonder we all resist. We bargain. We rationalize. We grieve. We get angry. Ultimately, however, if we want to lose weight, to lower our cholesterol levels, and to be healthy, most of us will have to make the change.

So the terms "balance" and "moderation" are ways to resist, bargain, and rationalize.

"Sure, you can eat a cheeseburger. Just balance it with lower-fat foods the rest of the day."

"Extra-sharp cheddar cheese melted over your broccoli? Sure. All of that fat can be balanced with lower-fat choices elsewhere in the meal."

And so it goes. The idea is that by balancing high-fat foods with low-fat foods, it all evens out and everything is fine. The reality, of course, is that most people don't do a good enough job of the balancing act. They eat too much of too many high-fat foods. They don't eat enough plant matter—fruit, grains, vegetables, legumes. Most importantly, though, by not making more fundamental changes in the way they eat, they perpetuate a way of life that undermines their dietary goals and their health.

With the trend in dietary recommendations toward a more plant-based diet, the concept of "variety" is a trump card played by many in the food industry and in certain nutrition circles. "Eat a variety of foods" is often followed by warnings not to "omit entire food groups." The danger here, of course, is that people might get it into their heads that meat, eggs, cheese, and other dairy products should be limited. That wouldn't be good for business for many in the food industry, nor for their friends.

When all is said and done, "no good foods, no bad foods" and "variety, balance, and moderation" are words that sound like advice but don't actually have a useful meaning. They don't step on toes, they don't offend. They're friendly, feel-good words that don't disappoint. They don't elicit change. They perpetuate the status quo.

 "If the health fanatics and obsessed nutritionists—the scareheads—succeed in taking over, they're going to kill gastronomy."
—Chef Julia Child, in a December 1994
interview for *Town and Country* magazine

Eating is One of Life's Greatest Pleasures

Or maybe gastronomy will change, as all things evolve and change over time. Is that so bad? Does it mean that food will never taste good again, or that a new way is going to spoil all the pleasure?

I love good food. Food brings me a great deal of pleasure. But I also eat healthfully.

My own family made the transition to a plant-based diet gradually in the 1970s. It took the full decade. With parents from Wisconsin, I was raised with the "heartland mentality" about food. I snacked on chunks of cream cheese and bowls of tapioca pudding made with whole milk. Mom's macaroni and cheese was my childhood favorite. But these and other traditions, such as the Easter ham and Thanksgiving turkey, faded away with time.

New traditions took root. Today, when my family gathers for Thanksgiving dinner, there simply isn't room on the table for a turkey—and nobody would want it, anyway. We've long since moved on to dishes like stuffed acorn squash and many-bean salad. The table is covered with hot whole-wheat yeast rolls, baked sweet potatoes, and fresh fruit salad. The table is a gorgeous, bright, festive display of healthful foods that taste great. Deprivation is the farthest thing from anyone's mind. Holiday meals are tremendous fun. They are also healthful.

Eating is one of life's greatest pleasures. Changes in dietary recommendations don't mean that the pleasure has to end.

But here's what's happening: Science is pointing to a diet that is outside our culture as being optimal for human health. In Western countries, meat and other animal products play a prominent—make that dominant—role in the diet. Ask a neighbor what he is going to have for dinner tonight and what is he likely to respond? A baked potato and a helping of green beans? Not likely. The answer will probably be "chicken" or "we're grilling steaks." The rest of the meal is of lesser importance. The meat is the focal point of the plate. The remainder of the meal is relegated to the side of the plate, in relatively small servings.

If we are to respond to the preponderance of scientific data on diet and disease relationships, then we have to discard old dietary paradigms and move toward a diet that is centered, instead, on foods of plant origin: fruits, vegetables, grains, legumes, nuts, and seeds. This is a diet in which meat, eggs, and dairy products play a very minor role, if we choose to eat them at all. And that's not American.

"American" is standing rib roasts and steaks cooked outdoors on the grill. "American" is macaroni and cheese and cake with ice cream, not lentil stew or vegetable curry over rice. "Don't mess with my traditions" is how some people feel.

Some people bristle at the thought of changing the way they eat, particularly if they feel that change is being foisted upon them.

A hilarious article in the February 1994 issue of *Spy* magazine posed the question, "How NC Are You?" How nutritionally correct, that is. The article chronicled what it termed the accelerating success of the "neoprohibitionist movement." It took jabs at "post-socialist outfits like Public Citizen and the Center for Science in the Public Interest" that want to "get the padlocks back on your pleasure chest." These "busybodies are busier than ever about our bodies."

The article points out that drinking alcohol at social functions has become nutritionally incorrect, thanks to the "neoprobes." At restaurants, "Ordering a mere beer is a minefield. Does he or doesn't he? What will she think of me? How many vegans are at this table?"

At the conclusion of the piece, the author notes that "nutritional correctness holds a pride of place in the media, in the Clinton administration and, alas, in an alarming number of kitchens. Not anymore. We say it's spinach, and we say to hell with it."

It seems that to resist change is to be human.

Give Me the Facts and Let Me Decide

A message that runs in *Good Medicine*, a newsletter published by the Physicians Committee for Responsible Medicine, reads:

"Last year, over a million people left the same suicide note."

Alongside the text is a picture of a hand-scrawled shopping list. On it are the words, "butter, eggs, mayo, potato chips, ham, bacon."

I know, I know. Some people can eat these artery-cloggers all their lives and live to be 100 years old. My own grandfather lived well into his 90s eating a low fiber, fat-laden diet.

No doubt many factors account for our health status at various stages throughout our lives. A select few of us may be genetically programmed to fare well despite a diet high in animal protein, cholesterol, and saturated fat. The vast majority of people, however, do not. Some people can get away with a poor diet, but I wouldn't bank on being the exception.

In fact, it appears clear now that even the conservative dietary guidelines that have been in place for many years—guidelines that have called for the public to limit fat intake to 30% of calories—don't result in dietary changes that are substantial enough to produce significant health benefits for most people. Research on patients with severe coronary artery disease has shown that those who follow the standard American Heart Association guidelines get worse, while those who limit fat intake to 10% of calories get better and show reversal of plaque buildup in their arteries.

The old recommendation of limiting fat intake to 30% of calories was political, in part, because it was largely a value judgment. Scientists chose this level partly because they felt that it was an attainable goal for most Americans whose usual fat intake was much higher. Researchers were afraid to set the level lower for fear that people would reject the recommendation outright. So rather than setting the goal at a level that was optimal for human health, the number was set at a level that scientists felt the public would accept.

Today, there is growing sentiment within the scientific community that dietary recommendations should reflect what is scientifically accurate, rather than what scientists think people will accept. There is abundant evidence to conclude that an optimal diet for humans is far lower in fat as compared to the traditional Western diet and is composed primarily of plant matter: fruits, vegetables, grains, legumes, and small amounts of seeds and nuts. The healthiest diets contain about 10% to 20% of calories from fat—depending upon the individual—and are very low in saturated fat, which comes primarily from animal sources. (Some individuals—particularly those who are at normal weight or have high calorie needs—can fare well on higher fat levels of up to 25% or 30% of calories from fat, as long as the saturated fat intake is very low.) Translated into real food, that means a diet that is generally low in fat and nearly or entirely vegetarian.

While not all people may choose to change the way they eat, most would probably agree that they are entitled to accurate information about what is best for their health. Give me the facts and let me decide what's right for me.

Putting the Politics into Perspective

The "politics" within groups of health professionals or government agencies are dynamic. Positions or statements made by organizations reflect what the current leadership thinks but may not be consistent with the opinions of some individuals or small groups within the organization. If those individuals and small groups persevere, they can eventually influence and change the voice of the organization as a whole.

For example, efforts to overhaul the national school lunch program

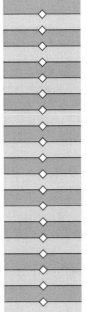

Viewpoint

"It is understandable and, in fact, perfectly reasonable that organizations such as the American Dietetic Association (ADA) adopt what may seem to be very 'conservative' positions on dietary issues. Nutrition is a very fickle field and rarely are data entirely consistent. That is why it is frequently so difficult to establish a scientific consensus. What must be avoided at all costs is for health agencies to continually rescind dietary recommendations. This leads to a loss of confidence among consumers which, in turn, can lead to consumer apathy about making dietary changes. For this reason, I think it is also best for all health professionals to err on the conservative side when making dietary recommendations. However, the often-conflicting scientific literature should not be used as a shield behind which organizations like the ADA can hide when the weight of the evidence dictates that dietary recommendations be made."

—Mark Messina, Ph.D.
Co-Author, *The Vegetarian Way* (Crown Books, 1996)

were launched within the USDA in the early- to mid-1990s. Proposed changes to school meal regulations called for requiring, for the first time, that the USDA comply with its own Dietary Guidelines in planning and monitoring school meals. In order to boost the fiber and reduce the fat and cholesterol content of school meals, these changes necessitated, among other things, a reduction in the use of high-fat commodities and high-fat meats and dairy products, the use of which the USDA had historically protected and promoted in looking out for industry interests.

There were individuals and groups within USDA that resisted these changes, but it was the efforts of some progressive groups and individuals within the same organization that made some changes possible. When all was said and done, the results of the overhaul of school meals appears to have been "two steps forward, one step back." The point is, however, that within this organization that has a history of protecting its industry interests, there exist individuals who are working instead to make public health a priority and take a different tack in their approach to implementing dietary recommendations.

Similar examples can be seen within groups of health professionals,

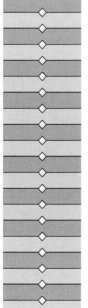

Viewpoint

"As the 16th-century French essayist Montaigne wrote: 'There were never in the world two opinions alike, any more than two hairs or two grains. Their most universal quality is diversity.' But our differences, whether they are religious, social, professional, or political, serve to make us more informed, to challenge us, and contribute to our personal and professional growth. Our differences give us a richer environment in which to learn from each other, to find our similarities, and to move our issues forward together.

"We are learning to listen to views that are antithetical to our own and to understand that there are many ways of seeing the same issue. Tolerance and acceptance of opposing views, various opinions, diverse cultural mores, and disparate values are essential to our multiculturalism."

—American Dietetic Association President Ronni Chernoff, Ph.D., R.D., F.A.D.A., in a discussion of the values of the American Dietetic Association, *Journal of the American Dietetic Association*, December 1996

such as the American Dietetic Association. The ADA leadership has a long history of protecting its relationships with industry groups, in part by not making any negative statements about particular foods. However, in recent years, a vegetarian nutrition dietetic practice group—a subgroup within the ADA—was organized by ADA members who want to explore nontraditional, plant-based diets. The practice group has worked to produce nutrition education materials that promote plant-based diets for the public and encourage people to consume fewer foods of animal origin. The group sponsors conference sessions at the ADA's annual meeting that focus on vegetarian diets, and the group produces a newsletter that is circulated among members.

The ADA is a large organization, and choices made by the leadership do not always speak for individual members or subgroups of the parent organization, some of which "politic" within the association for changes.

The point is, dietary recommendations are what they are, in part, because of politics. Because "politics" is the result of interactions among individuals and groups, the outcome is always changing. For now, though, you need to be aware of how the current political climate has influenced the dietary recommendations that you are hearing today. You need advice that has your best interests at heart—not the interests of industry groups or professional associations.

Let's peel back the layers of confusion produced by the politics of your plate and expose the truths behind recommendations about how you should eat.

Chapter Two

They Say, "Eat a Variety of Foods"

The 1995 edition of the USDA's Dietary Guidelines for Americans places the recommendation to "eat a variety of foods" at the top of its list, as it has since the inception of the guidelines in 1980.

The American Dietetic Association has publicly endorsed the guidelines.

They say, "Eat a variety of foods." What do they mean?

Foods contain a variety of nutrients, such as fiber, vitamins, minerals, protein, carbohydrate, and fat, as well as other substances. It's a good bet that there are many substances in foods that have not yet been identified but that are important for good health. That's why it's best to get what you need from whole foods, rather than relying on vitamin-mineral supplements. No single food contains everything you need. By eating a wide range of foods, you'll maximize the probability that you'll get the full spectrum of necessary nutrients.

By eating a wide variety of foods, you'll also dilute, in a sense, poten-

"What is the trait you most deplore in others?"
"Being an extremist of any sort."
"Which living person do you most despise?"
"An extremist of any kind."
"What is it that you most dislike?"
"Rigid, uncompromising, angry extremists."

—Chef Julia Child, in an interview
for *Vanity Fair* magazine, March 1996

tial negative consequences of a single food that may have some undesirable qualities. For instance, peanuts are rich in fiber, B vitamins, and Vitamin E, but if you ate nothing but peanuts, you would get too much fat in your diet, since peanuts are nearly all fat. By varying your food choices and including fruits, vegetables, and grains, you would decrease the proportion of fat your diet contains.

Another example might be if a food contained a toxic substance. By varying your food choices rather than eating primarily that particular food, you would minimize your exposure to the toxic substance. In that way, variety in your food choices can protect you.

Nutrients interact with each other. Some may even have a synergistic effect. Do you remember when beta carotene made headlines for its potential role in reducing the risks of cancer and heart disease? Vitamin companies began adding beta carotene to their supplements; beta carotene was even added to some brands of orange juice. Everyone was popping supplements of beta carotene. Then, later research found that supplements of beta carotene didn't seem to have the same protective effect as did whole foods that contained beta carotene.

There are over 600 carotenoids. Beta carotene is only one of them. Perhaps beta carotene works its magic in concert with other substances found in whole foods, or maybe it isn't the beta carotene at all but rather another substance that, by coincidence, happens to be found in foods that are rich in beta carotene. The moral of the story is to get the nutrition you need from whole foods, and include a wide range of foods in your diet.

But They Also Say...

So far so good. It's what comes next that is a problem. Discussion about the importance of eating a variety of foods is usually followed by the stipulation that to do so means choosing foods from "the major food groups" and the importance of "balance" among food groups in the daily diet. "Don't omit a whole food group," is a customary warning.

The evidence pointing to a plant-based diet as being optimal for humans is hard to ignore, so updated dietary recommendations now note that the diet should be comprised chiefly of servings from the "grain, vegetable, and fruit groups." Recommendations are to eat "moderately"

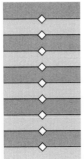

For the same number of calories as in three glasses of skim milk, you could eat any one of the following:

5 1/2 cups of steamed broccoli

9 carrots

1 2/3 cups of cooked oatmeal

1 1/3 cups of cooked kidney beans

2 1/2 medium bananas

(there's that word again) from the "milk and meat groups," and to choose fatty and sugary foods only sparingly.

"Moderate" consumption of meats and dairy products is defined in the Dietary Guidelines as two to three servings from the meat group and two to three servings from the milk group each day.

Therein lies the problem.

Meats and dairy products are the primary sources of saturated fat and cholesterol in the American diet. Even if low-fat varieties of these foods are chosen, these foods still contain cholesterol, are still devoid of fiber, and have high concentrations of protein. These foods are major sources of substances that Americans generally consume in excess. To recommend that people eat several servings of these foods each day means devoting a substantial portion of the diet to these foods. Conversely, it means that there is less room in the diet for health-supporting, fiber-rich plant products.

Think about it this way. Three servings of skim milk would provide about 270 calories. Imagine how much broccoli, carrots, oatmeal, beans, or bananas you could eat for the same number of calories.

You can guzzle a glass of milk down in no time. Since there's no fiber in milk, it isn't very filling.

If you passed up the milk, think of how much more plant matter you could eat for the same number of calories.

Think of how much fiber you could add to your diet. As a point of reference, the typical American consumes about 10 or 12 grams of fiber per day, while current recommendations encourage a minimum of 25 to 35 grams of fiber per day.

One three-ounce serving of lean meat contains about 165 calories. In reality, most people eat much more than three ounces of meat in a typical

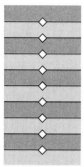

For the same number of calories as in three glasses of skim milk, you would get the following amounts of fiber from these foods:

milk—no fiber

oatmeal—7 g.

steamed broccoli—22 g.

carrots—10 g.

kidney beans—21 g.

bananas—4 g.

serving, and they do not choose the leanest varieties. Three ounces is less meat than in an average chicken breast.

Imagine eating two or three servings of meat per day. If you only ate two two-ounce servings of lean meat, it would contain about 220 calories. Two three-ounce servings of a medium-high-fat meat total about 450 calories. Most people eat even more than that.

Can you visualize how much fiber-rich plant matter you displace from your diet when you include the "recommended" moderate number of servings of meat and dairy products in your diet each day? Really, there's nothing "moderate" about it. It's too much.

So they say, "Eat a variety of foods," "Choose foods from the major food groups," and "Don't omit whole groups of foods." What they don't say is that there is a better way than the traditional American eating pattern. What they don't say is that it is far healthier to choose less meat and more beans from the "protein" group and that by reducing your overall intake of protein, you won't have to rely on quite so many servings from the "milk"

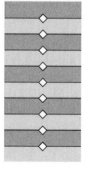

what's left to eat?

"Mediterranean is just the latest novelty resulting from America's fanaticism about calories and cholesterol and all that. The nutritionists and food press say that a regimen of vegetables and beans and pasta and olive oil is the ideal solution, and everyone gets on the bandwagon. I recently saw this so-called Mediterranean diet that allowed for no more than sixteen ounces of meat per month. That's insane!"

— Chef Julia Child

GOOD FOODS, BAD FOODS

group in order to meet your calcium needs.* In fact, there's no human "requirement" for milk in your diet at all past infancy.

What They Should Say Is...

"What about calcium? What about protein.... and iron?" you ask. Most of us are conditioned to think of animal products as the best or only sources of certain nutrients. Can you name a few foods that are rich in calcium? Most people would respond, "milk, yogurt, cheese." How about protein? Meat, fish, poultry, and eggs are probably the first foods that come to mind. Iron? Most people think of red meat.

In truth, dairy products are superconcentrated sources of calcium, and meat is a concentrated source of protein. Animal products such as these are ultra-rich sources of certain nutrients, but they aren't mandatory components of a healthy diet for humans. For a calf that needs to build a massive skeleton in a relatively short period of time, cow's milk is made to order. The physiology of a cat is such that large quantities of protein are needed, and meat supplies it in an efficient package. We humans have other sources of these nutrients, however, that are well suited to our unique needs.

Human beings, of course, have no requirement for milk from a cow. Milk is species specific. Dogs produce milk for puppies, cats produce milk for kittens, and cows produce milk for calves. Humans need human milk when they are infants, and in the next few years, they outgrow their need for it. So why the emphasis on drinking cow's milk for calcium? Even adult cows don't drink cow's milk.

In truth, calcium is widely available in foods of plant origin. Under ideal conditions (a world that didn't include fast food restaurants on every corner), we could get all of the calcium we needed from green, leafy vegeta-

---

*In the revised Dietary Guidelines for Americans, what used to be termed the "meat group" is now called the "meat and beans group", which is a step in the right direction. However, the fact that beans are a far better choice than meat is not revealed. These choices are essentially deemed equals, according to the Dietary Guidelines, especially if lean meats are chosen. In my experience, most nutritionists generally continue to recommend the inclusion of meat in the diet and are not comfortable advocating a diet without it.

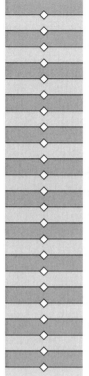

It's the Politics of Your Plate...

In 1994, the California Milk Advisory Board sent packets of materials to dietitians throughout the state, encouraging them to recommend dairy products to their Asian clients. The packets included instructions and educational materials designed to assist nutritionists in introducing dairy products into the diets of Asians, for whom dairy foods are not a tradition.

Asians, like many people who are not of Northern European descent, are typically lactose intolerant—fully 95% of Asians have some degree of lactose intolerance. (A genetic mutation that occurred thousands of years ago in Northern Europeans is thought to have made it possible for descendants to continue digesting milk into adulthood.)

People who are lactose intolerant suffer, to varying degrees, from gas, bloating, cramps, and diarrhea when they consume dairy products. Instead of pointing out the good sources of calcium that are already a part of the traditional, healthful Asian diet and encouraging Asians to eat plenty of these foods, the California Milk Advisory Board materials focused on the nutritional contributions of dairy products. It gave recommendations for introducing dairy products into Asian diets while minimizing the symptoms of lactose intolerance.

bles such as kale, collard greens, mustard greens, and a host of others. Broccoli, bok choy, dried beans and peas, dried figs, sesame seeds, and many other foods are good sources of calcium, too.

"But serving for serving, these foods have less calcium than dairy products contain. Won't I have to eat a truckload of broccoli in order to get what I need?"

The short answer is "no", but the explanation is much more complicated. Most people do need to pay attention to their calcium intake, but they don't have to drink milk.

The Recommended Dietary Allowance (RDA) for calcium is adjusted to meet the needs of people living the typical American lifestyle. That lifestyle includes dietary characteristics that increase our loss of calcium through the urine. One of those characteristics that I mentioned in Chapter 1 is an excessively high intake of protein. If you moderate your protein intake instead, you'll retain more calcium. The best way to moderate your protein

GOOD FOODS, BAD FOODS

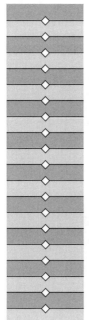

Do the White Thing?

While the California Milk Advisory Board may be focusing its efforts on getting Asians to drink milk, another campaign may be just as politically incorrect. In the award-winning "milk mustache" ads, many African American athletes and celebrities, including Spike Lee, Florence Griffith Joyner, and Tyra Banks, have been sporting their milky-white upper lips on billboards across the country, despite the fact that 75% of all African Americans are lactose intolerant.

Are these individuals inadvertently reinforcing ethnocentric dietary guidelines that encourage the consumption of cow's milk, even by those whose bodies can't tolerate it? Maybe Spike Lee and other African American celebrities should instead be promoting the consumption of soymilk, a nutritious alternative that would alleviate the suffering that comes from ingesting a food that the body is not equipped to handle. Asians, Native Americans, Jews, and Hispanics would also benefit from alternatives to cow's milk, since the majority of individuals in these ethnic groups are lactose intolerant to some degree.

intake is to eat less meat. Eat less meat, and you'll probably get more fiber in your diet, less saturated fat, and so on. So eating less meat is a good move for lots of reasons, including the fact that you'll hang on to more calcium.

Unfortunately, Americans also tend to consume large amounts of sodium, much of it in the form of sodium chloride, or table salt. Large intakes of sodium increase the loss of calcium from the body. Salty chips and snacks, soups, condiments such as ketchup and mustard, packaged mixes, and other processed foods all contribute to our high sodium intakes.

Phosphates in soft drinks may cause an additional loss of calcium, though not as significant as that from sodium and excessive amounts of protein. What's more, inadequate amounts of vitamin D—the sunshine vitamin—may also result in lower rates of calcium absorption.

We can make our own vitamin D by getting exposure to sunshine— about 15 minutes on face and hands at least three times a week. But some people don't make enough of it. They may live in smog-filled cities or in northern latitudes where there are fewer sunny days and where they work indoors or are housebound and rarely see the light of day. Plus, dark-skinned people need more sunlight than do light-skinned people.

Vitamin D, which helps your body absorb calcium, is generally not present in foods. The exception is dairy products, because they are fortified with vitamin D in the U.S. The amount of vitamin D that is present, however, is very unreliable and varies widely from one milk sample to another. Tests have shown that skim milk, in fact, has little if any vitamin D. The most reliable source of vitamin D is actually sunlight exposure or a supplement of not more than 100 percent of the RDA, since more can be toxic.

So, if you don't drink milk, do you have to eat a truckload of broccoli in order to get adequate amounts of calcium? That depends on all of the factors above and more, including whether you have a genetic risk for osteoporosis, which is the disease that weakens bones and allows them to break easily, especially in older women. People with a family history of osteoporosis need to pay particular attention to getting enough calcium in their diets, to eating a diet that will help them absorb and retain dietary calcium (less sodium, less protein, plenty of vitamin D), and even to other lifestyle factors, such as not smoking and getting plenty of weight-bearing exercise, which helps to keep bones strong.

Do Children Need Milk for Adequate Calcium?

Human infants need milk, and the best source is human breast milk. Commercial infant formula is an alternative when breast feeding is not an option. Babies need milk—but not cow's milk—for the first few years of life, until they are weaned and move on to table food.

What about afterwards? Do children need to drink cow's milk in order to get enough calcium? After all, children and teens are in a period of rapid

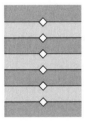

what's left to eat ?

"The only thing worse for your heart than fat is the stress generated by reading the relentless news reports about how just about everything we eat will kill us."

—*San Francisco Examiner* columnist *Bruce Bellingham*

GOOD FOODS, BAD FOODS

growth and development. During the first 30 or 35 years of age, in fact, humans are attaining "peak bone mass."

Although it is likely that people who moderate their protein and sodium intake actually need less calcium than those who eat a traditional American diet, the majority of scientific data that show this to be true come from people of other cultures who are eating plant-based diets. We, unfortunately, have little or no data about the calcium needs and bone health of young people eating plant-based diets in our own culture.

Therefore, it seems prudent for now to encourage young people to strive for meeting at least the RDA for calcium—an admittedly ambitious goal, because it is so high—just to be on the safe side. (In fact, a report issued in 1997 by the Institute of Medicine recently recommended increased intakes of calcium for U.S. and Canadian individuals and population groups, including children. The report was the first in a planned series of reports that will update and expand the current RDAs.)

But that doesn't have to mean drinking cow's milk. Young people who don't drink milk might be wise, though, to include some calcium-fortified foods in their diet, such as calcium-fortified soymilk or fortified orange juice. Cup for cup, these products contain just as much calcium as milk.

Additionally, they should aim for eating large servings (1 cup, cooked) of high-calcium vegetables such as dark greens—collard, kale, turnip, mustard—broccoli, bok choy, or legumes such as pinto beans, garbanzo beans, and kidney beans. The calcium from these foods, in fact, is absorbed by the body as well as or better than the calcium from dairy products. Three or four servings of any of these vegetables per day is a reasonable goal.

Big servings of vegetables are the order of the day on plant-based diets. Let's face it, a half-cup serving of anything isn't very much, so one-cup servings are not what I'd call overwhelmingly large. However, if you are young and you know that you do not consistently eat well, you might consider taking a calcium supplement to be on the safe side. Your health-care provider can discuss this with you.

The bottom line: if you avoid eating excessive quantities of protein, the amount of calcium that you'll need from your diet will be lower. You'll conserve even more calcium, however, if you moderate your sodium intake (see Chapter 6) and ensure that you are receiving (or producing) adequate amounts of vitamin D.

So if you ate nothing but foods of plant origin and no dairy products

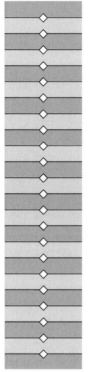

It's easy to get calcium from plant sources. For a calcium-rich dish, try:

Fresh kale sauteed with minced garlic and a drop of olive oil

Steamed broccoli with a squeeze of fresh lemon juice; sprinkle with slivered almonds

A stir-fry of bok choy, carrot coins, and cubed tofu (the kind that has been processed with calcium)

Mixed greens (mustard, collard, and turnip greens) sauteed with chopped onion, minced garlic, and a drop of olive oil; drizzle with your favorite type of vinegar

A bowl of many-bean chili (your choice: garbanzo, kidney, pinto, black, navy, and chili beans are a few ideas)

A tofu-salad sandwich (made with tofu processed with calcium)

A pita pocket filled with hummus, a delicious garbanzo bean spread; alfalfa sprouts; and chopped tomatoes

Winter salad made with chopped apples, oranges, and figs

Bean burritos or bean tacos

Bean tostada on a lime-processed corn tortilla

whatsoever, you might very well get less calcium in your diet than someone who drinks milk. But if your protein intake is moderate at the same time, and you watch your sodium intake and have plenty of vitamin D, then your lower calcium intake may be of no consequence. Studies from around the world, for instance, show that vegetarians who take in less than the RDA for calcium do not appear to have health problems as a result. They do not, as you might think, have higher rates of osteoporosis and may, in fact, have less osteoporosis.

It bears repeating that more research on Americans' eating vegetarian-style, dairy-free diets is needed, however, before anyone can say precisely what their calcium requirements may be. Therefore, it's best to err on the conservative side in this case and to encourage everyone to strive for close to the current RDA for calcium (which varies by age and sex; see Appendix). Those whose calcium needs are highest, such as children and young women, should take particular care to reduce their sodium intakes, to get adequate vitamin D, and to moderate their protein intakes.

GOOD FOODS, BAD FOODS

If the RDA for calcium is the goal, it is wise to try to get as much as possible from plant sources. If you choose to eat dairy products for their calcium content, they should be nonfat. Even then, they should be limited to about two servings per day so that they do not displace large amounts of fiber foods that provide so many essential nutrients and other health-promoting substances.

That means eating hefty servings of calcium-rich plant foods—one cup each of broccoli, greens, or cooked beans, for instance—three or four times a day. If you can't reach the RDA for calcium with plant foods alone, drink calcium-fortified orange juice or soymilk. You may also consider taking a calcium supplement, in which case your health care provider can advise you about how much and what kind to take.

The complicated issue of dietary calcium needs is wrapped up in value judgments about how Americans will choose to live and eat as well as limited by the small amount of research available on Americans eating other than the typical American diet.

And protein?

To get enough protein, all you have to do is get enough calories to meet your energy needs and eat a reasonable variety of foods of plant origin—vegetables, grains, and legumes. It's that simple.

It's easy to get enough protein from plant sources. Some protein-rich dishes include:

Vegetable stir-fry over steamed rice

Bean, lentil, or split-pea soup

Lentil and rice pilaf

Bean burritos and tacos

Vegetarian chili (serve over rice for a change of pace)

Pasta primavera

Vegetarian burger patty on a whole-grain bun

Large baked potato stuffed with mixed vegetables

Toasted pita points with black-bean dip

French bread pizzas made with tomato sauce and soy cheese

Fettuccine with pine nuts and basil

It's much the same story for iron. Although most people think of meat when they are asked to name an iron-rich food, plants contain plenty of iron as well. Plant foods that are good sources of iron include dark-green leafy vegetables, blackstrap molasses, dried fruits, prune juice, and many other foods.

Eating foods rich in vitamin C with meals helps the body to absorb the iron from plants. Citrus fruits and juices, tomatoes, cabbage, potatoes, and watermelon are a few vitamin C-rich foods. You probably eat foods rich in vitamin C with your meals and don't even realize it. Go easy on coffee and tea, though. They contain substances that can impair the body's absorption of iron.

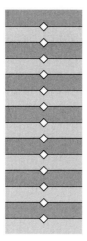

It's easy to get enough iron from plant sources. Some dishes or meals rich in both dietary iron and vitamin C are:

Steamed broccoli with a squeeze of fresh lemon juice

Spaghetti with tomato sauce

Iron-fortified breakfast cereal with a grapefruit half

Hot oatmeal with chopped, dried fruit and a glass of orange juice

Carrot, green pepper, and celery sticks with salsa and black bean dip

Black bean and corn salad topped with chopped tomatoes

Lentil soup with a mixed green salad and mandarin orange sections

Spinach salad with fresh strawberry halves

Setting the Record Straight

The fact is, it's wise to eat a variety of foods. It's just that the term "variety" doesn't mean you need to include several servings of dairy products and meats. You would actually be better off limiting the amount of dairy products and meats that you consume. You could choose to eat none at all. Protein, calcium, iron—you can get the nutrients you need from foods of plant origin (see The New Century Garden Guide, page 37.)

When dietary recommendations address the issue of variety, they should make it clear that the only foods that are basic to good health are foods of plant origin—fruits, vegetables, grains, legumes, and small

GOOD FOODS, BAD FOODS

amounts of nuts and seeds—foods that come from the soil. If, for reasons of personal preference, a person wants to include foods of animal origin such as meat, eggs, cheese, and other dairy products, then it should be clear that these foods are optional and are best limited.

Food Groups

The concept of food groups is somewhat arbitrary. The traditional four food groups—milk, meats, fruits and vegetables, and grains— were grouped that way because the foods in each group shared similar nutritional compositions. In reality, however, there is a great deal of overlap in nutrient compositions among all of these foods. Foods could be categorized in any number of ways.

Dr. T. Colin Campbell, a nutritional biochemist and director of the China Health Project at Cornell University, has a unique perspective on the issue. He prefers to speak of two food groups: plant foods and animal foods. "Eat a variety of stems and leaves and twigs and fruits and berries," he has said.

Recently, he has taken his concept further with the design of "The New Century Garden Guide." The seven sections of the guide represent different sections of the plant: leaves, roots, flowers, fruits, grains, legumes, and nuts. Eating a variety of these plant parts each day—at least five per day—will ensure that you get the range of nutrients that you need for good health.

———————————◇———————————

The New Century Garden Guide: Plant Parts and Their Nutrients*

Plant Part	Sources	Rich In
Legumes	Dried and fresh peas and beans	Magnesium, phosphorus, thiamine, iron, folate, vitamin K, protein, dietary fiber, carbohydrates
Grains	Corn, rice, wheat, rye	Magnesium, manganese, carbohydrates, protein, tocopherol (vitamin E), dietary fiber

*The nutrient lists could actually be expanded to show that, for instance, grains are also a source of thiamin and iron, and that flowers, nuts, leaves, fruits, and roots all provide fiber. Legumes, flowers, leaves, and some fruits contain calcium, and legumes, grains, nuts, and some fruits are also good sources of zinc.

Plant Part	Sources	Rich In
Nuts	Almonds, peanuts, cashews	Magnesium, copper, tocopherol, essential fats
Flowers	Broccoli, cauliflower, artichokes	Folate, vitamin C, vitamin K
Leaves	Lettuce, kale, swiss chard	Tocopherol, carotenoids, folate, vitamin C, vitamin K
Fruits	Oranges, peaches, tomatoes	Vitamin C, carbohydrates
Roots	Carrots, potatoes, yams	Carotenoids, vitamin C, carbohydrates

If you do choose to eat only foods of plant origin and to completely omit all foods of animal origin, you will need to have a reliable source of vitamin B12 in your diet. Vitamin B12-fortified breakfast cereals, fortified soymilk, or a vitamin B12 supplement (cyanocobalamin) are viable alternatives.

All animal products contain vitamin B12. However, while widespread in the soil, streams, and rivers (even produced in our intestines but beyond the site of absorption), there is none present in most of our plant foods per se. Some research shows that organically grown produce contains vitamin B12, but most Americans do not yet have easy access to affordable organically grown produce. And since we live in a sanitized society in which our fruits and vegetables are washed clean of soil and our water is chlorinated, we can't rely on these otherwise natural sources of vitamin B12.

Additionally, anyone who does not have adequate exposure to sunlight may need a vitamin D supplement. Your health care provider can help you determine whether your need for vitamin D should be assessed.

What You Need to Know Is...

It's a good idea to eat a variety of foods. Eat a range of fruits, vegetables (including plenty of green, leafy ones), whole-grain breads and cereals, and legumes, dried beans, and peas. Add some seeds and nuts, too (especially in children's diets, since they need more calories), but because they are high in fat and calories, use these foods only as a garnish or condiment.

GOOD FOODS, BAD FOODS

The greatest variety is in the plant world. There are literally hundreds, if not thousands, of different vegetables, fruits, grains, and legumes. Cultures around the world combine these foods in a myriad of ways to create delicious, nutritious meals.

When you hear nutritionists say "don't cut out whole groups of foods," they are usually referring to meats or dairy products. They are saying you should not omit meat or dairy products from your diet, since these foods are good sources of certain nutrients. They view the omission of these foods from the diet as "decreasing the variety" in the diet. They are wrong. The result is actually the opposite.

In truth, once you let go of the mindset that a meal has to center around a piece of meat, or that you need to eat two or three servings of dairy products every day, the variety in your diet will probably increase dramatically.

Think of it this way. How many different types of meats do you eat? Most people eat relatively few types of meat: beef, chicken, and fish, for the most part. How many ways do you prepare them?

As a practicing nutritionist, I've been hearing the "chicken and fish lament" for years.

"Chicken and fish. Chicken and fish. I'm overdosing on chicken and fish. What else can I eat besides chicken and fish?"

Fifteen years ago or so, when the public began catching on to the need to lower the fat and cholesterol levels in their diets, red meat consumption took a nosedive and bookstores exploded with cookbooks featuring 1,001 ways to cook chicken and fish the low-fat way.

Toss the chicken and fish aside, and you'll never have to complain about a monotonous diet again. Chapters 8 through 16 will help you get started.

You do not have to include meats and dairy products in your diet at all. If you do, the amounts should be limited and far less than what the standard American dietary guidelines suggest.

Dietary recommendations should point people to the diet that is the best possible way of eating for good health. The best possible way for you to eat is to make the vast majority of your food choices come from plant sources—much more so than traditional dietary guidelines issued in this country would suggest. Diets that contain no animal products at all can be nutritionally adequate and very healthful.

Most Americans need to increase radically the ratio of plant-to-animal products in their diets. See Chapter 14 for a meal-planning guide to help you get started.

Chapter Three

They Say, "Balance Your Food with Physical Activity"

Health professionals give exercise a great deal more attention now than they did in years past, especially when counseling people for weight control. I have distinct memories of the diet regimens of the 1960s and early 1970s, the years when the women of my mother's generation were trying to lose weight. The kind of exercise that was advocated then was little more than calisthenics—a few rounds of jumping jacks with Jack LaLanne. That same era gave us the dieter's special—a ground steak patty, a scoop of cottage cheese, a lettuce leaf, and slice of tomato for color. "I'll have a cheeseburger, hold the bun." That era.

People practically had to starve themselves to lose weight. They counted calories and munched on celery sticks and melba toast. Starches were "bad" and protein was king. Dietary fat was still an innocent, and slide aerobics and Nautilus circuits were not yet a part of the vernacular.

That's not to say that we have all of the answers yet. Weight control is

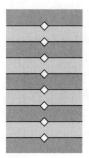

"Another good reducing exercise consists in placing both hands against the table edge and pushing back."

—Robert Quillen

"Often one or two low-fat cookies are not enough. 'What they don't tell you is that they eat the whole box instead of three or four cookies.'"

—*The Wall Street Journal*, November 20, 1996, in an article titled "Fattening of America: Less is No More" still a major heartache for a sizable segment of the population. But we're way past jumping jacks and fear of bread.

Instead, the importance of physical activity in controlling weight is widely recognized now, with the emphasis on a mix of vigorous aerobic activity coupled with anaerobic exercises for strength-building. Together, these types of activities help burn off extra calories, build muscle mass, and increase metabolic rate—all changes that make it easier to maintain an ideal weight.

Being physically active not only helps you stay trim, it makes it easier to be well nourished, too. The more active you are, the more food energy you need. The more you eat, the more likely you are to get all the nutrients you need. A couch potato who tries to lose weight on a 1,000-calorie diet is likely to have a tough time fitting adequate fiber and nutrition into such a meager calorie allotment. On the other hand, someone who steps up their physical activity and manages to lose weight while consuming 1,500 calories per day is more likely to meet his or her nutritional needs, as well as being less hungry and a lot happier.

For most of us, the key to successfully controlling our weight is to balance physical activity with the amount of calories we take in. Sounds like a simple enough proposition. But it's the translation of that simple concept into practical terms that leaves most people stuck in the mud, wheels spinning, going nowhere fast.

How so? It's a case of nutrition doublespeak as well as a little bit of soft-shoe. Standard recommendations dance around the real issues and avoid some important points that people need to know in order to make effective changes in their lifestyles.

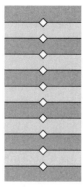

William Castelli, M.D., director of the Framingham Heart Study, commented on a "Sears Roebuck" approach to healthful eating, with these grades of quality:

"Good probably is the Mediterranean diet," with an emphasis on grains, fruits, and vegetables, with fat mostly from olive oil. Better is a low-fat diet, and better than low-fat is low-fat and vegetarian. That combination is hard to beat: The health record of vegetarian societies shows they outlive us and only have a fraction of our disease."

—from the *Chicago Tribune*, Sept. 1, 1994

But They Also Say...

Everyone agrees that weight control and general wellness require balancing physical activity with calorie intake. For most people, the physical activity should to be at least moderate in intensity, at least 30 minutes in duration per session, and frequent—you should exercise most days of the week.

But what about the food you eat? The kinds and amounts of foods you eat and drink have a major impact on your ability to control your weight. Which foods are best? Which foods should be limited? If I want to control my weight while eating enough of the right foods to stay healthy, what is the best diet?

The experts generally won't tell you—not precisely. You'll see the ol' softshoe when it comes to talking specifics about food. As I explained in Chapters 1 and 2, there is a strong value common in American nutrition circles that dictates that "there are no good foods and no bad foods" and that anything can be eaten in moderation. There is also an unspoken rule that says the system will support the traditional American eating style. This is perpetuated, in part, because of the political and economic interests involved.

All of these factors are reflected in the 1995 Dietary Guidelines for Americans, in which seven keys are highlighted for decreasing calorie intake by diet. They include:

- Eat a variety of foods that are low in calories and high in nutrients— check the Nutrition Facts Label.
- Eat less fat and fewer high-fat foods.
- Eat smaller portions and limit second helpings of foods high in fat and calories.
- Eat more vegetables and fruits without fats and sugars added in preparation or at the table.
- Eat pasta, rice, breads, and cereals without fats and sugars added in preparation or at the table.
- Eat less sugars and fewer sweets (like candy, cookies, cakes, soda).
- Drink less or no alcohol.

What is notable is not so much what is said—the points are all valid. It's what is not said that is significant and problematic.

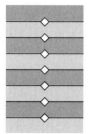

While many people have switched from whole to low-fat milk and from butter to margarine, and trimmed their appetite for red meat, Americans have also substantially increased their consumption of sugary soft drinks; also, they're eating more chicken, but a lot of it is fried. Call it the American paradox: Sales of high-fat premium ice cream are rising, and so are sales of low-fat yogurt.

—*The Wall Street Journal*, June 28, 1996

What They Should Say Is...

Fat is a concentrated source of calories. Gram for gram, fat provides more than double the number of calories as carbohydrate and protein. That means foods that are high in fat are the most concentrated in calories. If you want to control your weight, you need to minimize your intake of fat and fatty foods. On the other hand, foods that are rich in carbohydrate and low in fat tend to be bulky and filling. By eating plenty of low-fat, carbohydrate-rich foods, you'll tend to get full before you take in more calories than you need. It's the optimal way of eating for most of us, and it's Nature's way of keeping things in balance and your weight in control.

Unfortunately, the traditional American diet is loaded with fat. Most of it comes from meat and dairy products, followed by fats that we add to our foods, such as salad dressing, margarine, and oil used in frying. Have you heard the saying, "Worry about the dollars and not the pennies?" If Americans could cut down drastically on their intakes of the foods that are the biggest contributors of fat in the diet, calorie intakes would be reduced, and so would waistlines.

When fat intake decreases, fiber intake usually increases. The fiber comes from the grains, fruits, and vegetables that are eaten in place of the fatty meats and dairy products. Cutting down on the fattiest foods in the diet—meats and dairy products—is the way to "worry about the dollars." You'll get the biggest return for your effort.

The guidelines don't point this out. They name names, but only up to a point. They say to eat more fruits, vegetables, pasta, rice, breads, and cereals. They say to eat less sugar and fewer sweets, and they name names, specifying candy, cookies, cakes, and soda. But when it comes to the most powerful recommendation of all, addressed near the top of the list, they go mute. "Eat less fat and fewer high-fat foods" and "Eat smaller portions and limit second helpings of foods high in fat." Which foods are those?

What the experts won't say is that you should cut back on meats and dairy products, the biggest sources of fat in the American diet, in order to help you control your weight.

Small portions of these fatty foods are densely packed with calories:

3.5 oz. sirloin steak	352 calories
1 bratwurst link	256 calories
1 beef hot dog	180 calories
1 link pork sausage	265 calories
3 oz. McDonald's hamburger	263 calories
1 oz. cheddar cheese	114 calories
1 oz. (1 slice) American cheese	106 calories
1/2 cup Häagen-Dazs ice cream, butter pecan	310 calories
1 Tbsp. bleu cheese dressing	85 calories
1 tsp. butter	36 calories
1 tsp. corn oil	40 calories

These bulky, low-fat foods have relatively few calories in generous-sized servings:

1 medium apple	81 calories
1 cup blueberries	82 calories
1 medium kiwifruit	46 calories
1 medium mango	135 calories
1 medium orange	65 calories
1 cup cooked spaghetti	159 calories
2/3 cup cooked oatmeal	109 calories
3/4 cup bran flakes	93 calories
3 cups plain popcorn	69 calories
1 cup boiled asparagus	44 calories
1 cup boiled beet slices	52 calories
1 cup raw broccoli florets	24 calories
1 medium raw carrot	31 calories
1 cup cooked collard greens	27 calories
1 cup boiled green beans	44 calories

Do You Like to Eat? A Little or a Lot?

Long-standing, "don't ruffle anyone's feathers" guidelines to limit fat intake to 30% of calories also complicate people's efforts at weight control.

Do you remember the old Weight Watchers' meals of years past? The meal plans were based on a diet that derived 30% of its calories from fat, 20% from protein, and 50% from carbohydrate. Meals were American-style and usually built around a meat entree.

On a 1,000- or 1,200-calorie diet, a typical dinner consisted of a chicken breast cooked without the skin, a small serving of a vegetable, a slice of bread or other starch, and perhaps a small tossed salad with lemon juice or one teaspoon of regular dressing (this was before the days of commercial fat-free salad dressings). There might have been a piece of fruit for dessert or a small serving of canned fruit packed in water.

Can you visualize this meal on a plate? It isn't much. Small servings of vegetables, grains, and fruits were really small. The standard half-cup serving is only a few forksful. When your exercise regime consisted mainly of a few rounds of jumping jacks and you followed traditional dietary patterns, you didn't get much to eat. A lot of people walked around gnawing on their knuckles or surreptitiously raiding the cupboards.

I don't know about you, but I have a big appetite. I like to eat what I want to eat, and I don't like to worry about how much. That's why I stay physically active—the more active I am, the more calories I need for energy and the more I can eat. I'm not a marathon runner or elite athlete, though, so there's a limit to the number of calories that I can count on burning through exercise.

That's why I like to eat a low-fat, plant-based diet. By centering my diet on grains, fruits, and vegetables and limiting foods of animal origin, my dietary fat intake doesn't exceed 20% of calories, and I get to eat a whole lot more than I would if my diet was higher in fat and planned around a piece of meat. By loading up my plate with foods of plant origin, my diet is more varied, higher in fiber, and lower in fat.

I eat BIG servings of vegetables, and BIG servings of fruit. The truth is, there isn't room on my plate for a piece of meat. Fatty dairy products? They're only an occasional addition to a meal as a condiment—a sprinkling of Parmesan cheese over a salad or a smidgen of light cream cheese on a bagel.

I eat a greater volume of food and don't go hungry. Coupled with a habit of frequent, moderate to vigorous exercise, a typical dinner for me might look like this:

- A large mixed green salad topped with one cup of garbanzo beans, shredded carrots, a few black olives, ground black pepper, and a splash of raspberry vinegar;
- A large baked sweet potato topped with brown sugar and fresh lime juice;
- A toasted whole-wheat English muffin with jam;
- Half a cantaloupe for dessert.

These lifestyle habits—regular, almost daily, exercise and a low-fat, plant-based diet—allow me to enjoy a wonderful variety of delicious foods, and I can eat according to my appetite. I eat freely, I find great pleasure in my meals, I feel good, and as an added bonus, I find it relatively easy to maintain an ideal weight.

What You Need to Know Is...

You need moderate to vigorous physical activity almost every day. You'll feel better if you do, and you'll be able to eat a lot more food. Nobody likes to worry about what or how much they eat, and you won't have to if you stay active enough.

If you are starting from ground zero, you should realize that it takes time to establish a routine of physical activity. Once your level of fitness improves, it will take less effort to maintain it. It may be helpful to consult an exercise physiologist or personal trainer to get you started.

Your attitude toward exercise is critical to your success at establishing a routine that you can maintain for the long haul. You've got to enjoy what you're doing. Nobody said that an exercise routine had to consist of walking on a treadmill in your home or riding a stationary bike at the gym. Mix it up. Include a variety of activities that suit your personality and lifestyle. Your activities might depend upon the season, your schedule, or whether or not your kids are in school during the day. They can be costly and involve memberships to gyms or purchasing expensive equipment, or they can be free. It's your choice.

Exercise shouldn't be a prescription that you fill grudgingly. Ideally, being physically active is a value and lifestyle habit that is associated with pleasure.

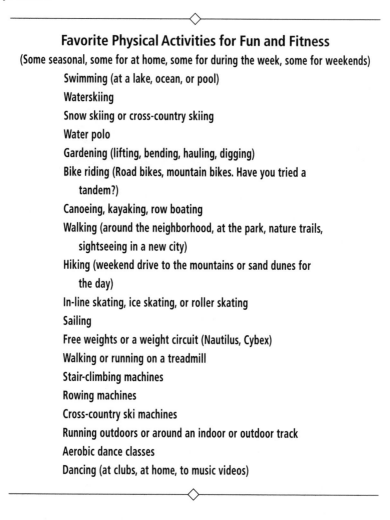

———————————◇———————————

Favorite Physical Activities for Fun and Fitness
(Some seasonal, some for at home, some for during the week, some for weekends)

Swimming (at a lake, ocean, or pool)

Waterskiing

Snow skiing or cross-country skiing

Water polo

Gardening (lifting, bending, hauling, digging)

Bike riding (Road bikes, mountain bikes. Have you tried a tandem?)

Canoeing, kayaking, row boating

Walking (around the neighborhood, at the park, nature trails, sightseeing in a new city)

Hiking (weekend drive to the mountains or sand dunes for the day)

In-line skating, ice skating, or roller skating

Sailing

Free weights or a weight circuit (Nautilus, Cybex)

Walking or running on a treadmill

Stair-climbing machines

Rowing machines

Cross-country ski machines

Running outdoors or around an indoor or outdoor track

Aerobic dance classes

Dancing (at clubs, at home, to music videos)

———————————◇———————————

It's easier to find a balance between physical activity level and diet if your diet is low-fat and plant-based. That means moving away from meat-centered meals and meals that include fatty dairy products. If you eat meats, they should be nothing more than minor ingredients in the dishes that you eat. They should be side dishes or condiments, rather than the focal point of the meal. The less meat the better.

Ditto for dairy. If you include dairy products in your diet, make them a condiment. Smear a little light cream cheese on a bagel if you must, or add a little grated Asiago cheese to your pasta. Plan to get your calcium from big servings of green leafy vegetables, broccoli, kidney beans and other favorite legumes, fortified orange juice, or any of the many other plant sources. Go back to Chapter 1 for more detail about dietary calcium requirements.

Cut down on added fats in your diet, such as oil, margarine, butter, and salad dressings. Read more about fats in Chapter 5.

Smart Snacks

Between-meal snacks can be fine when they are part of a lifestyle that includes regular physical activity and a low-fat, plant-based diet. Some good choices include:

Bean tacos and bean burritos

Baby carrots dipped in salsa

Fresh fruit—try seasonal fresh fruits, a frozen banana or
   frozen grapes, or an exotic fruit such as mango or papaya
   for a change of pace

Frozen fruit bars

Whole-grain cereal with skim milk or a low-fat nondairy milk
   substitute such as soymilk or rice milk

Bagel with jam

Homemade reduced-fat whole-grain muffins

Homemade reduced-fat oatmeal cookies

Four-bean salad marinated in oil-free dressing

A whole tomato in season, eaten like an apple

Applesauce with cinnamon

A baked apple with cinnamon and sugar

A big bowl of oil-free-vinaigrette cole slaw

Toasted English muffin with honey or jam

For more assistance with individual weight loss goals, consult a registered dietitian or other health care provider who is familiar with plant-based diets. The American Dietetic Association has a referral service that can help you identify practitioners in your area who have expertise in plant-based or vegetarian diets. Persons with this orientation will be the most helpful to you. The ADA's referral service can be reached by calling (800) 366-1655.

You may also find a suitable practitioner by word of mouth in your own community or through a referral by a member of a local vegetarian society. Also, see the resource list in Chapter 13.

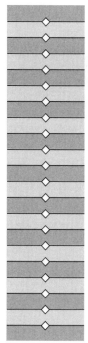

What About Weight Control For Kids?

Children need more calories than adults, due to their rapid rates of growth and development, so they can tolerate more fat in their diets than adults. While adults may fare well on diets with 10 to 20% of calories from fat, children may need up to 25% of calories from fat.

Many American children eat far more fat than this, and are also inactive; they spend too much time in front of the TV and playing video games rather than being active outdoors. As a result, obesity is a major public health problem for today's young people.

Children should eat the same low-fat, plant-based meals as their parents, and additional fat from plant sources such as peanut butter, avocado, and almond butter, or a few drops of olive oil on a salad can be added for extra calories. Children should also make physical activities a part of their daily routine. A tradition of regular family outings that are oriented to physical activities such as hiking, bike riding, or swimming will help to establish health-supporting habits early in life.

See the resource list beginning on page 148 for more information about nutrition for children and teens.

They Say, "Choose a Diet with Plenty of Grains, Vegetables, and Fruits"

Mom has been vindicated. Along with cutting down on fat, "Eat your vegetables" has emerged as the nutritional battle cry for our time. The national "5 a Day" campaign, which strives to motivate everyone to eat at least five servings of fruits and vegetables each day, has been endorsed by numerous health organizations. The campaign is a collaboration between the Produce for Better Health Foundation—a project of the fruit and vegetable industry—and the National Cancer Institute.

Since when did fruits and vegetables command so much respect? After all, it wasn't long ago that the old "Basic Four Food Groups" model for meal planning allocated a full 50% of the picture—two groups—to meats and dairy products, muscling out foods of plant origin, leaving one slot for breads and cereal products, and squashing the fruits and vegetables into a group of their own.

The fruits and veggies are finally pushing back, breaking out of the confines of a single slot and joining forces with the breads and cereals to overtake the animal products. The USDA released its new and improved graphic model for meal planning, the Food Guide Pyramid, which replaced the

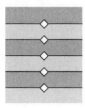

"Quite frankly, low-fat is one of those things that customers talk about, but it's not something they do."
— Allan Huston, president and chief executive of Pizza Hut, upon the restaurant chain's introduction of the TripleDecker pizza with 400 calories and 17 grams of fat per slice

Basic Four, in 1992. Since then, most health organizations have espoused the idea that the diet should be comprised mainly of grains, fruits, and vegetables, which make up the wide base of the Food Guide Pyramid (below).

They say to choose a diet with plenty of grains, vegetables, and fruits. Why?

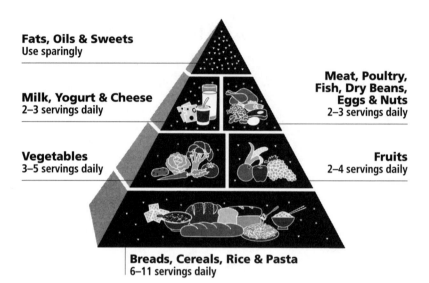

Fats, Oils & Sweets
Use sparingly

Milk, Yogurt & Cheese
2–3 servings daily

Meat, Poultry, Fish, Dry Beans, Eggs & Nuts
2–3 servings daily

Vegetables
3–5 servings daily

Fruits
2–4 servings daily

Breads, Cereals, Rice & Pasta
6–11 servings daily

The Fiber Factor

Fiber is one reason. But did you know that dietary fiber was once considered a food contaminant?

Not too long ago, dietary fiber was called "roughage" and was thought by many to be hard and irritating to the lining of the stomach. In the late 1970s and early 1980s, I recall working as a clinical dietitian and counseling hospital patients to eat more fiber. Some of them would say that they couldn't eat lettuce because it seemed scratchy and might bother their stomachs.

Funny. Just the opposite is true. Foods that are high in dietary fiber absorb moisture as they move through the gastrointestinal system and become soft and spongy, making stools larger and easier to pass and decreasing the pressure in the intestines. People who get plenty of fiber in

GOOD FOODS, BAD FOODS

their diets have fewer problems with constipation, hemorrhoids, diverticulosis, and diverticulitis. Large, soft stools require less force to pass, resulting in a decreased incidence of hiatal hernia and varicose veins in the legs.

Dr. Ken Heaton of the Department of Medicine, University of Bristol, Bristol Royal Infirmary in Bristol, UK, noting that diets of soft foods are associated with constipation and that fiber-rich diets are associated with a low incidence of constipation, coined the phrase "hard in and soft out" or "soft in and hard out." (From: *Western Diseases: Their Dietary Prevention and Reversibility.* Edited by: N.J. Temple and D.P. Burkitt. Humana Press, Totowa, N.J., 1994.)

It was people's early contempt for "roughage", however, that spurred the development of ways to extract fiber from grains by milling techniques that produced white, refined flour and, ultimately, Wonder Bread. We've come full-circle, though, and today, dietary fiber holds a place of honor in nutrition science.

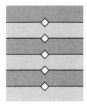 **Instead of giving up chocolate chip cookies for nutritious fruit and grains, for example, many people opt for popular low-fat brands like SnackWell's, and imagine that they are health conscious.**

—*The New York Times*, November 20, 1996, in an article titled "Fattening of America: Less is No More," written by Donna St. George

Fiber Has Many Talents

Dietary fiber not only adds bulk to the stool and prevents constipation, but it plays other health-supporting roles as well. Dietary fiber takes several forms. Some dietary fiber helps to slow the absorption of glucose into the bloodstream after a meal and can, for instance, help to control blood sugar levels in diabetics. The same form of fiber helps to lower blood cholesterol levels.

People who eat diets high in fiber have lower rates of colon cancer. An added advantage to eating a diet high in fiber is that environmental contaminants such as pesticide and herbicide residues that may be found in the food supply are moved through the body relatively quickly and have less time to be in contact with the lining of the gastrointestinal tract.

It's important to realize that fiber takes more than one form, though. Dietary fiber includes pectins, gums, cellulose, and hemicellulose, all with different functions in your body. Fiber supplements generally single out only one type of fiber. You need more for good health. Plan to get your fiber from whole foods and plenty of them. BIG servings of fruits and vegetables. BIG servings of grains. By eating a range of whole grains, fruits, and vegetables, you'll ensure that you'll get what you need.

But Wait... There's More

Plant matter is important for many reasons. Most fruits and vegetables are low in fat, high in fiber, and packed with vitamins and minerals. Recently, however, it has also been recognized that plant matter contains other substances—many not previously identified or given much attention—that play important roles in health promotion and disease prevention. These substances are called phytochemicals ("phyto" meaning "plant"), and there are thousands of them.

Examples of phytochemicals include isoflavonoids, such as genistein and daidzein, which are found in soy foods and act as weak phytoestrogens and may decrease the risk of breast cancer in women. A substantial body of research suggests that plant estrogens such as these may lower the risk of coronary artery disease, cancer, and osteoporosis, and may even relieve the hot flashes associated with menopause. Just the tip of the iceberg. Suffice it to say, foods of plant origin are full of substances that support health and may be useful in the prevention of chronic, degenerative diseases and other conditions.

What They Won't Say Is...

Conventional dietary recommendations now say to make the bulk of the diet whole grains, fruits, and vegetables. There's a piece of the picture missing, though. What they don't say is vital to a clear understanding of the dietary changes that need to be made.

I remember some of my first experiences as a clinical dietitian in hospitals, when I had to give discharge dietary instructions to patients. Invariably, I would receive my orders to provide nutrition counseling to the patient only moments before the patient was ready to leave. Usually, I'd arrive at a patient's room to find him or her dressed, perched on the end of the bed, bags packed, and ready to bolt out the door. I had just enough time to convey a few words of wisdom, hand the patient a "diet sheet"—usually a one- or two-page list of do's and don'ts—and wave good-bye. Sometimes I didn't even have that much time and had to run down the hall, chasing someone who was leaving by wheelchair, and push a diet sheet into his or her hand as he or she was wheeled away. "Call me if you have questions!"

A very common order was for a high-fiber diet instruction. The diet sheet that patients were given listed various high-fiber foods that should be included in the diet. The usual advice was to eat whole-grain bread, to choose whole-grain and bran cereals, and to eat lots of fruits and vegetables. It always struck me as odd that the instructions didn't mention that it would be especially helpful if those foods replaced low-fiber foods. Patients were left with the impression that they should add some high-fiber foods to their diet on top of the food they usually ate.

It's the same way with current dietary recommendations to eat more plant matter. What they won't say is that to make the bulk of the diet come from plant matter, you have to simultaneously eat fewer animal products. In other words, there's a second part to the standard recommendation. "Make the bulk of your diet come from grains, fruits, and vegetables" and do this by making animal products a smaller part of your diet.

There's no other way to do it. There's a limit to how much a plate can hold and how many calories you need. If the bulk of your diet is going to come from foods of plant origin, then those foods will have to displace foods of animal origin. Since animal products traditionally play a major role in the American diet and take up a lot of space on the plate, it should be made clear that this is tradition that needs to be changed.

But We Hate to Name Names

Mom may have been right when she said to eat your vegetables, but she also said, "If you can't say something nice, don't say anything at all." For the conventional nutrition community, it's politically taboo to suggest that meat or dairy consumption should be decreased. There are simply no bad foods.

The reluctance of mainstream American nutritionists to admit that some foods are better than others does a terrible disservice to the public and undermines community health and nutrition education goals. Once again, if dietary recommendations are going to paint a realistic picture of a health-supporting diet, then they can't stop short of a complete explanation.

When the statement is made that "Fiber is only found in plant foods like whole-grain breads and cereals, beans and peas, and other vegetables and fruits" as the 1995 Dietary Guidelines note, they should also point out that animal products such as meats, cheese, milk, and yogurt contain none. Only then will people begin to understand the extent to which their eating habits must change if they are to realize significant health benefits.

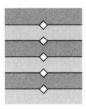

"And, of course, there are those folks who describe, say, fettuccine Alfredo as 'heart attack on a plate.' I wish people would take a more adult point of view, not feel so scared of things. Then they could eat sensibly and enjoy their food."

— Chef Julia Child

What You Need to Know Is...

The vast majority of the foods you eat should be from plant sources, as close to their natural state as possible. That means you should eat a variety of fruits, vegetables—including legumes such as beans and peas—and whole-grain breads and cereals. Your meals should be built around these foods.

At the same time, reduce your intake of animal products. Move away from meat-centered meals, and reduce your dependence on dairy products (see Chapter 15 for more help). The fewer animal products, the better. If you include animal products in your diet, make them minor ingredients in a dish, a condiment, or a side dish. Part Two of this book will help you get started.

"You Are Here"

Another way to express the way in which most Americans need to change their diets is to say that there should be a radical increase in the ratio of plant-to-animal products in the diet. Look at the graphs on the next page to see a graphic representation of that change.

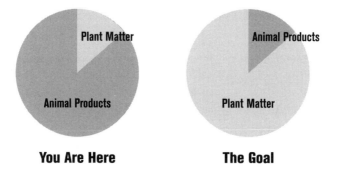

You Are Here   **The Goal**

Most Americans eat too many animal products and not enough plant matter.

Aim for at least 30 grams of fiber from whole foods every day. While it's not necessary to walk around with a calculator in your pocket, it doesn't hurt to have a goal in mind. If you are able to get at least 30 grams of fiber each day from whole foods (as opposed to fiber supplements), then it's a pretty good bet that you'll be getting adequate amounts of plant matter in your diet.

Take a look at the nutrition labels on foods you buy to check how much fiber they provide in one serving. Notice the size of the serving, as well. You might eat more or less. For instance, if the nutrition label on a box of cereal states that 3/4 cup of cereal contains 4 grams of fiber, and you eat twice that amount for breakfast, then your bowl of cereal provides you with 8 grams of fiber.

Spot check your fiber intake now and then by running a tally for a few days. Get the fiber information from food labels, or estimate the fiber content of other foods. The table on page 58 will give you an idea of the amount of fiber contained in some familiar foods.

There's no need to stop at 30 grams of fiber per day. If you consume more fiber than that, it's great. At one time, it was thought that "large" (a relative term!) amounts of fiber from foods could impair the body's ability to absorb minerals from your diet. That is no longer considered to be a problem, however. In fact, findings from the China Health Project, a large-scale population study of 6,500 people in the People's Republic of China, showed that intakes of fiber of as much as 77 grams per day caused no adverse effects.

Psst. Just Between Us...

If you currently eat a diet that is low in fiber and begin to dramatically increase your fiber intake, you may notice some increased flatulence, or gas. Not everybody finds this to be the case, and there's nothing dangerous about it—just a little inconvenient or potentially embarrassing. You may notice some gas pains. Flatulence tends to subside over time as your body adjusts to the increased fiber load. Being physically active helps to alleviate problems with flatulence, too.

Fiber Content in Grams of Some Common Foods

Fruits (1 medium piece or 1/2 cup canned)

Apple	3
Banana	2
Blueberries (1 cup)	3
Cantaloupe chunks (1 cup)	1
Fruit cocktail	1
Figs (4)	13
Grapefruit half	2
Mango	5
Orange	3
Papaya	1
Peach	1
Pear	4
Raspberries (1 cup)	6
Strawberries (1 cup)	4
Watermelon cubes (1 cup)	1

Vegetables (1 cup raw or 1/2 cup cooked)

Asparagus	1
Broccoli	2
Cabbage	2
Garbanzo beans (canned)	6
Green beans	1
Kale	2
Kidney beans (canned)	6
Lima beans	6

	Fiber (g)
Mustard greens	1
Swiss chard	1
Tomato	2
Winter squash	3
Grains and Grain Products (1/2 cup cooked or as specified)	
Bagel, 1 cinnamon raisin	1
Bran flakes, 1 cup	6
Bran muffin	3
Bread, one slice whole-wheat	3
Pita bread	1
Mixed-grain hot cereal	2
Oatmeal	2
Pasta	2
Rice, white	1
Rice, brown	2
Shredded Wheat, 1 cup	4

―――――――――――――◇―――――――――――――

Water, Too

Pay attention to how much fluid you drink, as well. The old "rule of thumb" recommendation to drink eight glasses of water a day is a reasonable goal. While you don't necessarily have to limit yourself to water, water is always the best choice. Flavored seltzer waters, fruit juice (many people like to mix it with mineral water or seltzer water), and vegetable juice are also good choices. The fiber in your intestines will absorb some of this fluid and help to make your stools soft and easy to pass.

If you don't want to count cups of water, just make it a habit to take frequent drinks during the course of the day. Each time you pass the kitchen sink, take a quick drink. When you pass a drinking fountain away from home, have a sip. Keep a tumbler full of water at your desk at work and a bottle of water beside you in your car, as well.

They Say, "Choose a Diet Low in Fat, Saturated Fat, and Cholesterol"

I hear it often. In response to admonitions about dietary fat and as a way of rationalizing that pint of Ben and Jerry's Double Chocolate Chunk, people will often remark, "Everyone needs some fat in their diets."

Yes, they do. You need about 5% of the calories in your diet to come from fat in order to provide you with enough of the essential fatty acids. That's actually a wee little bit of fat, though, and all of it can be gotten in the vegetables and grains that you eat, without fat having to be added to your foods and without the need to include high-fat foods in your diet.

Not that you can't include some high-fat foods in your diet. After all, getting only 5% of the calories in your diet from fat isn't the ultimate goal. A diet that derives 15 to 20% of its calories from fat is the best target for most people. Even at that level, however, there isn't a lot of extra room for high-fat items such as fatty meats, cheeses, and other high-fat dairy products, oils, margarine, and other added fats.

You might not have realized that there is fat in most vegetables and grains. A slice of bread, a bowl of oatmeal with nothing on it, and a half-cup serving of plain corn each contain about 2 grams of fat (where do you

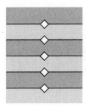

"There's no sound reason why we shouldn't be allowed to enjoy, say, six tablespoons of butter per day. After all, fats are fuels that fight disease, so to deprive your veins of all cholesterol is just asking for trouble the nervous Nellies don't tell you about."

— Chef Julia Child

think corn oil comes from?). Seeds and nuts are high in fat, which is why peanut butter and sesame tahini are so fatty. Avocados and olives are also nearly all fat. About the only way you could avoid fat in your diet altogether would be if you ate nothing but fruit, which is fat-free. Not recommended, as you might have guessed.

We only need about 5% of our calories from fat, but it's the extras I've already mentioned—the meats and dairy products that contain animal fats, the butter, margarine, and salad dressing, and the oil we fry with—that push our fat intakes to 20%, 25%, 30% of our calories and beyond. Considering how easily fat sneaks into our diets, and considering that fat is inherent even in grains and vegetables, there isn't much chance that anyone of us is going to be fat deprived, even on the most prudent of diets.

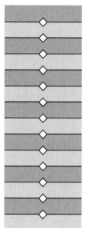

Jim stated that he, like every other American above the age of 4, is on a low-fat diet, and he noted that we have become basically a nonfat nation. This is true; virtually all edible substances, and many automotive products, are now marketed as being low-fat or fat-free. Americans are obsessed with fat content.

DOCTOR: Mrs. Stoatbonker, you will die within hours unless you take this antibiotic.

PATIENT: Is it fat-free?

DOCTOR: I don't know.

PATIENT: I'll just have a Diet Pepsi.

—Syndicated columnist Dave Barry in
"Nation's diet puts fat in fight for its life," 1996

The Landslide Case Against the Big Three: Total Fat, Saturated Fat, and Cholesterol

By now, most everyone knows that high intakes of total dietary fat, saturated fat, and cholesterol are linked with increased rates of coronary artery disease, some types of cancer, obesity, and other diseases and conditions. Despite the fact that this information has been available for many years now, and despite some improvements in the way that many people eat, most people are still eating far too much of the "big three." Why is that?

GOOD FOODS, BAD FOODS

What They Won't Say Is...

By now, you're getting the idea that, often, it's what is not said that is vital to an understanding of the issue. In the case of your diet, what is not said may be the missing link between hearing the recommendations and your ability to put those recommendations into practice. While not all people are motivated to change their eating habits for health reasons, some people would like to but haven't done so yet because they don't understand what to do.

When nutritionists say, "eat less fat, saturated fat, and cholesterol" and choose fewer foods that are high in these substances, they rarely, if ever, mention that this means eating fewer animal products. That's because of the unspoken rule that says people must be allowed to continue eating the traditional meat-centered, dairy-heavy diet. If meats and high-fat dairy products are mentioned, they are usually sandwiched between a litany of other fatty items, such as salad dressings, oil, margarine, nuts, and other fatty foods.

Meats and dairy products aren't singled out as being particularly troublesome. And they should be. Why? Because they are the biggest contributors to most peoples' intakes of total fat, saturated fat, and cholesterol.

There are many foods that contribute these substances in excess in our diets, but not to the extent that meat and dairy products do. Want to worry about the dollars and not the pennies? Want to get the biggest return for your efforts? Then move away from meat-centered meals, and cut down on your use of dairy products. If you don't make these most basic of changes, then it will be very difficult to make changes in your diet that are substantial enough to result in significant health benefits.

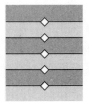
"The fries were fine when they cooked them in beef tallow, but then the nutrition police got in on the act and insisted on hydrogenated vegetable oil. Now the potatoes have no flavor whatsoever. I do think, however, that they'll soon come back to their senses."

— Chef Julia Child

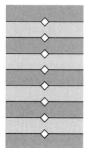

First, however, we need to consider exactly what fat is. Just off the top of my head, without glancing at a dictionary, I would define fat as "any of various mixtures of solid or semisolid triglycerides found in adipose animal tissue or in the seeds of plants." A triglyceride, as I vaguely recall from my high-school years, is "any of a group of esters, CH2(OOCR1) CH(OOCR2)CH2(OOCR3), derived from glycerol and three fatty acid radicals.

—Columnist Dave Barry, 1996

Trimming the Fat

Of course, another reason that you may have found it difficult to make effective changes in your eating habits is that a primary criterion for those changes has been inaccurate. Mainstream recommendations to limit fat to 30% of calories don't go far enough to produce significant health benefits, as I discussed in Chapter 1.

The decision to designate 30% of calories from fat as the goal was a value judgment—a political decision—rather than one based on science. The unfortunate result has been that a tremendous amount of energy, time, and money have been poured into programs and educational materials that hold 30% as the target—a "moderate" goal—and one that falls short of that needed to improve health.

In fact, research directed by Dean Ornish, M.D., of the Preventive Medicine Research Institute, found that when people with severe coronary artery disease followed a vegetarian diet and reduced the fat in their diets to 10% of calories, they were able to reverse the buildup of plaque in their arteries and halt the progression of their disease. On the other hand, those people who followed the standard American Heart Association guidelines, which called for dietary fat to be limited to 30% of calories, got worse.

A continuation of Dr. Ornish's research has shown that the longer people follow a low-fat, plant-based diet, the greater the reversal of their disease. Findings from this research suggest that eating a vegetarian diet and limiting dietary fat to 15% of calories may prevent the onset of coronary artery disease, while limiting fat intake to 10% of calories may reverse existing disease. A non-vegetarian diet with a dietary fat content of 30% of calories almost guarantees that coronary artery disease will progress.

What They Should Say Is...

It bears repeating: What they should say is that the most effective way for most people to reduce the total fat, saturated fat, and cholesterol in their diets is to move away from meat-centered meals and to eat fewer dairy products. Information about how to make the transition to a more plant-based diet is supplied in Chapters 8 through 16.

They should also pair the terms "low-fat" and "plant-based" in order to give the most accurate picture of how a health-supporting diet should be planned. Just choosing low-fat options from the various food groups, without regard for the other nutritional features of the food, doesn't necessarily mean that dietary needs will be met.

How so? Consider a few examples.

Some people, in only considering the fat content of foods, substitute fat-free cheese for full-fat cheese, nonfat ice cream for regular ice cream, and skim milk for whole milk. They may choose hot dogs that are 98 percent fat-free in lieu of a regular brand, and they buy fat-free cold cuts to make sandwiches instead of buying the old-fashioned, greasy kind. They buy fat-free sour cream, fat-free cream cheese, fat-free whipped topping, fat-free mayonnaise, fat-free you-name-it.

In making these substitutions, they have cut back on the fat in their diets, which is good. However, they have also replaced one animal product with another. In doing so, they did not increase the ratio of plant-to-animal matter in their diet. They did nothing to boost their fiber intakes. Nor did they increase their intakes of beneficial phytochemicals that they may have gotten by substituting a plant product for an animal product instead. And they were probably still left with diets that were excessively high in protein.

In that sense, worrying only about the fat content of your food choices can be a red herring. It can distract you from other, more comprehensive changes that you need to make. Not only should you consider the fat content of foods, but you should choose foods that are plant-based as well as low in fat.

Instead of piling a sandwich high with fat-free cheese and fat-free cold cuts, for instance, why not have one skinny slice of a flavorful, low-fat cheese and then pile the sandwich high with grated carrots, spinach leaves, and tomato and onion slices? Or skip the cheese altogether and add a tablespoon or two of a good chutney for flavor, instead. Or swap a fat-free hot dog for one of the many delicious vegetarian burger patties on the market made with combinations of beans, rice, vegetables, or soy protein, or try a vegetarian hot dog product instead.

Put Total Fat and Type of Fat in Perspective

Very-low-fat vegetarian diets are associated with a reduction in the risk of coronary artery disease, but it's most likely because these diets are low in saturated fat and cholesterol. It's possible that plant-based diets that are higher in fat—but not excessively high in fat—would produce the same results.

That may be why populations seen in other parts of the world, such as the Mediterranean, have lower rates of heart disease despite higher fat intakes. The fat that they eat comes primarily from plant sources and is monounsaturated, as in olive oil. Their intakes of saturated fat and cholesterol are comparatively low.

The reason a fat intake of approximately 15 to 20% of calories—as opposed to 30% or higher—is probably optimal for Americans is that a lower fat intake helps with weight control and allows for the bulk of the diet to come from unprocessed plant foods. Then, in addition to keeping the total intake of fat low, it's also important to keep saturated fat and cholesterol intakes low in order to reduce risk of coronary artery disease.

Since cholesterol is found only in animal foods (and even very lean meats can be high in cholesterol), and since saturated fat is found primarily in foods of animal origin, the best way to avoid saturated fat and cholesterol is to greatly limit animal products. Processed foods, such as commercial baked goods and snack foods, can also be high in saturated fat, so it's a good idea to limit them as well.

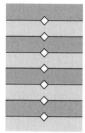

what's left to eat?

"The low-fat-cookbook business has become a bloated and distended juggernaut that threatens to crush everything else on the market."
— Jeffrey Steingarten, in an article for *Vogue* magazine, in which he laments the onslaught of recipes that trade "real food" ingredients for flavorless, fat-free substitutes that don't deliver

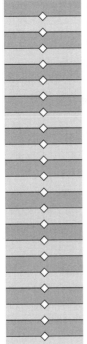

Of course, there have been efforts to make low-fat "hamburgers." In researching this column, I purchased a product called "Harvest Burgers," which are "All Vegetable Protein Patties" manufactured by the Green Giant Corp.

... the key ingredient in Harvest Burgers is soy. This ingredient is found in many low-fat foods, and I think it's time that the Food and Drug Administration told us just what the hell it is. A plant? A mineral? An animal? Are there enormous soy ranches in Nebraska, with vast herds of soys bleating and suckling their young? As a consumer, I'd like some answers. I don't want to discover years from now that soy is an oriental word meaning "compressed ant parts." This is not intended as a criticism of the "Harvest Burger," which is a well-constructed, extremely cylindrical frozen unit of brown foodlike substance. The package states that it contains "83% less fat than ground beef"; I believe this, because it also tastes exactly 83% less good than ground beef. Nevertheless I highly recommend it for anybody who needs more soy or a backup hockey puck.

—Columnist Dave Barry, 1996

What You Need to Know Is...

You should choose a diet low in total fat, saturated fat, and cholesterol by centering meals around grains, fruits, and vegetables instead of meats and dairy products. Meats and dairy products contribute the lion's share of fat, saturated fat, and cholesterol in most people's diets. Minimize your intake of these foods, and you will have taken the most important step in improving your diet.

Additionally, added fats such as salad dressings, oils, margarine, butter, fat used in frying, and so on should also be limited or avoided altogether. There are other foods that are also high in fat, such as nuts and seeds, avocados, and olives, but your use of these foods can be addressed, if needed, in "fine-tuning" your diet later. First things first. For now, worry about the big steps, the steps that will give you the biggest return for your effort.

Limit your intake of fat to about 15 or 20% of the calories in your diet, particularly if you are striving for weight control. This is prudent advice for most people. Do this by increasing the ratio of plant-to-animal products in your diet. Again, your meals should be based on grains, fruits, and vegetables with little or no fat added. Meats and dairy products, if included in the diet at all, should be present only on the order of a condiment, a side dish, or a minor ingredient in a dish.

Once again, the caveat here concerns the possibility that some individuals may do fine on higher fat intakes, providing that the fat is from plant sources and is primarily monounsaturated.

Remember that most dietary recommendations are recommendations for groups of people, not for individuals. As an individual, your particular situation and needs may be different. If you are physically active and have no trouble keeping your weight at a healthy level, and you eat a plant-based diet that is higher in fat—for instance, up to about 30% of calories from fat—that may be fine.

Also, there is evidence that people with existing coronary artery disease can reverse their disease by eating a vegetarian diet with only 10% of calories from fat (in conjunction with stress reduction, moderate exercise, and smoking cessation), but it's likely that weight control and limitation of saturated fat and cholesterol are the dietary factors responsible for these results.

No Need for Calculators, But...

If it helps you to have a more specific goal in mind, then try this: On a 15% fat diet, someone who needs 1,500 calories per day should limit his or her fat intake to about 25 grams per day. A 20% fat level would equal 33 grams of fat per day.

An 1,800-calorie diet? About 30 grams a day for 15% fat, 40 grams on a 20% fat diet.

For a 2,000-calorie diet, limit fat to about 33 grams per day for a 15% fat diet, or 44 grams for 20% fat.

On a 2,500-calorie diet, limit fat to about 42 grams per day for a 15% fat diet, or 56 grams for 20% fat.

When you read food labels at the supermarket, remember that the "goals" that are noted on the label are set using the standard of 30% of calories from fat. That's too much fat for most of us. Ignore this information and focus instead on the actual number of grams of fat per serving in the product. The actual number will give you a good enough idea of how the food fits into your diet.

For instance, if the nutrition label on a frozen entree states that one serving contains 14 grams of fat, and your "budget" is 25 grams of fat per day, then you can see that this item would contain more than half of the fat you should eat in a day. An entree that contained 5 grams of fat in a serving would be more reasonable.

Pocket "fat counter" books available in any bookstore will give you the fat contents of foods without labels. While I am generally not an advocate of "counting" nutrients in foods on a daily basis, I understand that it helps some people to stay on track.

If you enjoy or need this kind of approach, then the two most important nutritional features to look for are fat and fiber. In very general terms, most people can aim for 30 grams of fiber per day or more and 30 grams of fat per day or less. If you can keep your fiber intake high and your fat intake low, most other aspects of your diet will fall into place as well, as I'll discuss in more detail in the next chapter.

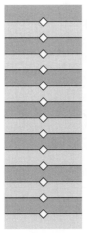

What's left to eat?

Oh sure, there will be people who will claim that soy patties taste "almost as good" as real hamburgers. These are the same people who have convinced themselves that rice cakes taste "almost as good" as potato chips, when in fact eating rice cakes is like chewing on a foam coffee cup, only less filling. You could fill a container with roofing shingles and put it in the supermarket with a sign that said "ZERO-FAT ROOFING SHINGLES," and these people would buy it and convince themselves it tasted "almost as good" as French toast.

—Columnist Dave Barry, 1996

As for Saturated Fat...

Conventional recommendations for saturated fat intake generally call for not more than 10% of total fat intake to come from saturated fat. In its most recently revised dietary guidelines, for instance, the American Heart Association recommends limiting saturated fat intake to 8 to 10% of total fat intake. Patients following Dr. Ornish's heart disease reversal program had saturated fat intakes of only about 2% of their total fat intakes. A figure somewhere in between—around 6 or 7% of total fat— is probably reasonable for most people. That translates to about 2 grams of saturated fat on a 1,500-calorie, 20% fat diet, or about 3 grams of saturated fat on a 2,000-calorie, 20% fat diet.

Should you count grams of saturated fat, total fat, or both? My advice: Don't drive yourself nuts wielding a calculator every where you go. Focus on the "big picture" recommendations that I've provided, including generally watching your intake of total fat and dietary fiber (without necessarily "counting" it), and stick to a diet that is plant-based, as we've discussed. You'll get close enough to your goal, and you'll preserve your sanity, too.

Chapter Six

◇ **what's left to eat?**

They Say, "Choose a Diet Moderate in Sugar, Salt, and Sodium"

Fat, saturated fat, cholesterol, sugar, salt, sodium, pesticides, herbicides, food additives—with so many dietary no-no's, it's no wonder some people throw up their hands and cry, "Uncle!" How is anyone supposed to find anything to eat?

Sometimes it all seems so complicated. Actually, the science of nutrition is complicated, but being well-nourished is a relatively simple matter. Have you ever had a huge project to complete or a large volume of information to learn? What seems overwhelming at first glance can seem more manageable when taken in smaller pieces. Breaking a project up into several smaller components, and focusing on completing one component at a time, can reduce the stress and boost your spirits.

You can use the same strategy in handling matters of nutrition and your diet. In this chapter, we'll look at ways to organize and prioritize your dietary goals. But first, here is some background about some of the dietary no-no's that may be sending you over the edge:

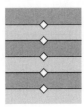

"Pesticides are a red herring for the public. Worry about the bigger issues, such as fat—there's a bigger return for the effort. You can drive yourself nuts worrying about every aspect of your diet."
—Robert Pritikin, director of the Pritikin Longevity Centers, Santa Monica, Calif.

Sugar

Just a spoonful helps the medicine go down. A little bit in your oatmeal tastes good, too.

Most people think of table sugar, or sucrose, when they hear the word "sugar." But sugar actually comes in many forms. Honey, fructose, molasses, syrup (corn syrup, maple syrup, rice syrup), Turbinado or raw sugar, brown sugar, glucose, dextrose, maltose, and others are all forms of sugar you may see listed on food labels. One isn't better or worse for you than the other. As far as your body is concerned, sugar is sugar.

Sugars are carbohydrates, just like dietary fiber and starches. Dietary fiber and starch are considered "complex" carbohydrates and take longer to break down during digestion than sugars. Sugars are considered "simple" carbohydrates and are digested more quickly. Although dietary fiber is only partially digested at best, both starch and sugar are eventually broken down into glucose, the simplest form of sugar. The glucose is then absorbed into your bloodstream and used for energy. Your body stores some sugar in your muscles, too, but excess calories from sugar are converted and stored as fat.

You may not have realized that, just as some foods contain starch, many foods also contain simple sugars. These naturally occurring sugars can be found in breads and cereals, milk, fruits, and vegetables. Just as everyone needs some fat in their diet, we also need some sugar. But just like we don't actually have to add fat to our diets to get what we need, we also don't have to eat table sugar to get enough. Just eating a wholesome diet containing grains, fruits, vegetables, and legumes provides all of the sugar you need.

On the other hand, most of us like to add sugar to our foods. We love its sweetness and the way it makes other foods taste. In fact, we also like foods that are primarily sugar. We love candy, soft drinks, and sweet desserts. Most of these are "empty-calorie" foods, which means they don't provide you with much in the way of nutrition in exchange for the calories.

If you are a super-athlete and burn up hundreds of extra calories a day, then a few sweet treats on top of an already-healthful diet are probably not an issue. But for most of us ordinary folk, a couple of soft drinks or a candy bar each day means "empty-calorie" junk foods are displacing more healthful foods that provide much-needed nutrients, especially vitamins, minerals, and fiber.

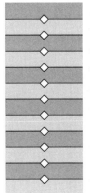

Calories Count

The latest chapter in the fat trap is the proliferation of fat-free desserts. Can you have your coffee cake and eat it, too? Not necessarily. Despite the fact that there are now many fat-free cakes, cookies, brownies, and other treats on the market, most people don't have carte blanche to eat all they want. Since these foods tend to be highly processed, fiber-less, and high in sugar, a small serving can add up to big calories. If you are watching your weight, watch out for these foods. If you can't stop at one slice or two cookies, you may be better off leaving these out of your grocery basket.

Sugar Substitutes

Sugar substitutes come in many forms. Sugar alcohols, such as mannitol and sorbitol, are used in chewing gum, toothpaste, and some sugar-free candies. Some people get diarrhea when they eat a huge quantity of sugar alcohol-sweetened food, but this type of sweetener has otherwise not been associated with health concerns.

Aspartame, which is marketed under the brand names of Equal and Nutrasweet, is made from two amino acids, which are components of protein. It's used in a variety of sugar-free foods, including soft drinks, drink mixes, gelatin and pudding mixes, candy, and many others. The government has deemed aspartame to be safe for most people (with the exception of children with a condition known as PKU), although some consumer groups have concerns due to case studies of people who have complained of neurological symptoms (such as headaches) after consuming aspartame-sweetened foods.

Saccharin, known by many people as Sprinkle Sweet, Sugar Twin, and Sweet N' Low, is an artificial sweetener that has long been used in soft drinks and a host of sugar-free food products. It has been shown to be a mild carcinogen, causing bladder cancer in laboratory rats. Concluding that the risk to people is small, the government has sanctioned saccharin for use by the general public, but food products that contain it must display a warning label—much like that on a pack of cigarettes—stating that the substance has been shown to cause bladder cancer in rats. In other words, use this product at your own risk. Nobody really knows what minimal exposure to a carcinogen is necessary before cancer will result. Environmental factors may also play a role and act synergistically with a carcinogen such as saccharin to produce a tumor.

Salt and Sodium

Sodium is a mineral that occurs naturally in foods. Some of these foods are higher in sodium than others, and the same food can even vary in its sodium content depending upon where it is grown. Just like fat and sugar, we all need some sodium in our diets. But the amount we need is very small, and we can get all we need from what is naturally present in food without adding it.

The most common way that people add sodium to their diets is the use of table salt, or sodium chloride. Salty or high-sodium condiments such as soy sauce, ketchup, mustard, commercial salad dressings, and others also add large amounts of sodium to our diets. We get even more sodium in processed foods. Frozen dinners, packaged mixes, soups, cheese, snack chips, and many other foods can be loaded with sodium. Salt or sodium-containing substances are added to foods to enhance the flavor of foods or as a preservative.

Your taste or preference for salt is acquired, which means you can condition yourself to prefer less saltiness. Have you ever tasted low-sodium tomato juice or low-sodium soup? If so, you probably thought it was exceedingly bland. But if you avoided salt and high-sodium foods for a length of time—weeks for some people, months for others—your taste buds would adjust. The next time you ate a salty food, it would probably taste overbearingly salty.

Salt Substitutes

At the supermarket, you may have seen the "light salt" and salt substitute on the shelf next to the regular table salt. Whereas table salt is sodium chloride, salt substitute is a salt made with potassium—it's potassium chloride. It has a salty taste but leaves a bit of a bitter aftertaste. "Light salt" is a mixture of table salt and salt substitute, or half potassium chloride and half sodium chloride.

What's Wrong With Salt?

High intakes of sodium are associated with higher rates of hypertension, or high blood pressure. People with a predisposition for high blood pressure can reduce their chances of developing the disease if they limit their intake of salt and high-sodium foods. High intakes of sodium may also increase the body's loss of calcium through the urine. Salt substitutes—potassium chloride—don't have the same effect, although people with certain medical conditions such as kidney disease may have to avoid potassium chloride as well.

Additives, Preservatives, Pesticides, and Other Environmental Contaminants

The mainstream nutrition community has, in general, not given much attention to the issues of undesirable food additives and environmental contaminants such as herbicides and pesticides. This may be largely due to the fact that there are other more pressing issues with which to contend—fat, cholesterol, fiber, salt, sugar.

But it may also be because the government has deemed safe the food additives about which some individuals and consumer groups have concerns. Large, national food producers generally do not use organic farming techniques, so organically grown foods are not readily available in some communities. When they are, they often cost much more than conventionally grown products.

How should you handle these issues? Read on.

What They Won't Say Is...

Whether they take the finger-wagging approach ("Don't eat this, don't eat that") or an ambiguous, positive tack, American Dietetic Association-style ("Any food can fit into a healthful eating style"), health professionals make it clear that there are many aspects of your diet that you have to think about: fat, saturated fat, cholesterol, fiber, variety, balance, sugar, and salt.

You may hear about still others—additives, environmental contaminants—through the media, consumer groups, and other organizations.

What you won't hear is practical advice about how to organize and prioritize these dietary issues. That's too bad, because for all the effort and money that go into the development and dissemination of nutrition and health messages, if people don't know how to put the recommendations into practice, then they can't easily meet goals for dietary change. And all of these dietary issues do have to put into perspective in order for anyone to get a handle on how to go about making changes.

What You Need to Know Is...

Worry about the dollars and not the pennies. You've heard this advice before, but it's an extremely important point that will help you to organize your goals, prioritize, and perhaps save your sanity.

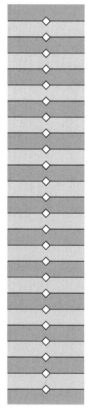

It's The Politics of Your Plate...

Not long ago, any self-respecting nutritionist routinely recommended only 100% juice when counseling clients or writing menus. Juice "drinks," as they were called, were blends of fruit juice and sugar water and were looked upon with disdain. Juice drinks were considered inferior to 100% juice because the 100% juice was more nutritious. It contained more vitamins, minerals, and who-knows-what-yet-to-be-identified other substances that are necessary for good health.

A few years ago, the American Dietetic Association declared that it had taken a new stance on the subject. The Association now judged the nutritional composition of juice drinks to be the same as for 100% juices, and that either was an appropriate choice.

In November 1995, *The New York Times,* in an article by Marian Burros titled, "Additives in Food Advice?" reported that "After receiving a $70,000 grant from Ocean Spray Cranberries, Inc., the [ADA] help line ran a message that said some juices, like cranberry juice, must be blended to make them drinkable, but still compared favorably in nutrition with 100% juice."

In this case, the scientific facts surrounding the issue had not changed; what had changed was the Association's way of looking at them.

The most important dietary pointers are to keep fat intake low and fiber intake high, and to radically increase the ratio of plant-to -animal products in your diet. These are the changes that will give you the biggest return for your effort. Not only do they address the most significant dietary issues, but if you make these changes, then other dietary factors (sugar, sodium, and so on) will more easily fall into place. That's because plant foods that are low in fat and high in fiber tend to be less processed, lower in sodium, and less likely to have sweeteners added.

That's not to say that issues such as sugar and sodium are not important. They are. But most people do best making gradual changes in their diets, a step at a time. Once you've mastered the biggest, most fundamental changes, then you can fine-tune your diet by turning your attention to the remaining issues.

Again, focus on the big items first—fat and fiber, more plant matter, and fewer animal products. Once you've mastered these changes, then you can think about fine-tuning.

Eat foods that are as close to their natural state as possible. The closer a food is to its natural state, the less likely it is to contain added sodium, sugar, and undesirable additives. Foods that are less processed usually contain more fiber, too.

About Organics

I try to buy organically grown fruits and vegetables when possible in order to minimize my exposure to environmental contaminants such as pesticides and herbicides. I especially like to buy locally grown produce when it's in season. Sometimes I find it at the farmers' market or at roadside stands.

But I often do not buy organic foods. At the supermarket, organically grown foods can be far more expensive than other foods. (Hopefully that will change someday as organically grown food becomes more popular and widely available.) And while I expect to find a few blemishes on my organic produce, sometimes I find that organically grown produce at the supermarket has begun to spoil because it doesn't sell as fast as less expensive non-organic foods.

If I don't buy organic, I wash my produce with a little dish soap and water, and I peel anything that has a waxy coating on it.

However, one of the advantages of eating a plant-based diet is that most foods of plant origin contain only a small fraction of the amount of environmental contaminants that are found in meats and dairy products. Environmental contaminants are concentrated in animal tissues. Minimize your intake of animal products, and you minimize your exposure to these contaminants.

A low-fat, plant-based diet also decreases the amount of time it takes for foods to work their way through your body. If your diet is high in fiber, contaminants will be less likely to be absorbed and will move more quickly through your system. Fiber may also bind some contaminants and help remove them from your body. For these reasons, I don't get overly concerned when it isn't practical for me to buy organically grown foods.

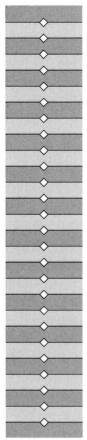

Learn New Skills One Step at a Time

As a teen, I was a competitive swimmer. My experience learning proper swimming techniques taught me how to tackle complicated new skills one step at a time.

I had to learn four different swimming strokes: the backstroke, the breast stroke, the butterfly, and freestyle. For each stroke, there was a string of points to remember. "Chin back, hips up, thumb at 2 o'clock, rotate your shoulders but keep your head still, kick the water up all the way to the ceiling...." At least 10 things to remember for each stroke.

Had my swim coach expected me to master all 10 points right away, I would have been immobilized and sunk. Instead, during daily workouts, he had me swim 20 laps of each stroke over and over again, focusing on one or two ideas for each stroke that I practiced. Later, after I had perfected those first techniques, it was time to add a couple more. And so it went, until the basic techniques became second nature. At that point, I would swim laps while my coach watched from poolside, barking out commands that amounted to fine-tuning my style.

By systematically learning the techniques of swimming, I acquired skills that have remained with me all of my life. Like swimming, changing your eating habits takes time and effort. Taking changes a few at a time helps ensure that you are not overwhelmed at the outset and that you master fundamental changes before moving on. One step builds on another.

About Sugar and Salt

Foods that are in their natural state are usually low in sugar and sodium. Fresh fruits and vegetables, whole grains, and dried beans and peas, for instance, have no sugar or salt added. All they contain is what nature gave them. These are the most wholesome foods.

The best policy is to limit sweets and salty or high-sodium foods. For most people, though, it's fine to eat these foods occasionally if they are used as condiments. Condiments are products added sparingly to enhance the flavor of foods. Salty or sweet condiments may be especially worthwhile if they replace a fatty condiment. You are better off, for instance, using a teaspoon of mustard (high in sodium) on a sandwich instead of adding mayonnaise (all fat). You are better off putting a teaspoon of jelly on a piece of toast (sweet) rather than a teaspoon of margarine (all fat).

It's okay for most people, for instance, to add a couple teaspoons of brown sugar to a bowl of oatmeal. The little bit of sweetener makes a bland bowl of oatmeal more enjoyable for most folks. It's okay, too, to drizzle a little honey over a bowl of bran flakes or shredded wheat. It's much better than eating a refined, presweetened breakfast cereal or eating a donut or breakfast pastry.

Another example: Instead of a munching on a bag of salty chips, try dipping carrot sticks (low in sodium) into salsa (a condiment that is often salty) for a snack. A smidgen of mustard (salty) on a tomato sandwich (low in sodium) is fine for most people and is a better choice than eating a sandwich that is piled with high-sodium cheese.

Of course, there are many reduced-sugar and low-sodium food products, including condiments, on the market now, and these can be good choices. If you would like more help in choosing the healthiest foods at your supermarket, my book *Shopping for Health: A Nutritionist's Aisle-By-Aisle Guide to Smart, Low-Fat Choices at the Supermarket* may be useful to you.

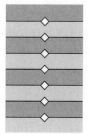 "Here's a hot tip: buy the low-sodium V-8 juice and add a little Tabasco sauce to it. I always add a little Thai hot sauce, particularly if I'm eating a low-sodium soup, or a squeeze of lemon. It brings out the flavor without adding sodium."

—Robert Pritikin, director of the Pritikin Longevity Centers, in the book, *Shopping for Health: A Nutritionist's Aisle-By-Aisle Guide to Smart, Low-fat Choices at the Supermarket*

Remember: focus your energy first on fat, fiber, and plant vs. animal matter in your diet. Once you've mastered these changes, then you can fine-tune by reducing sodium and sugar.

About Sugar and Salt Substitutes

You'll need to use your own judgment in deciding whether to use sugar substitutes such as aspartame or saccharin, and whether to use salt substitute. Decisions pro or con are based more on value judgment than on science.

I personally try to avoid sugar substitutes and prefer to use small amounts of the real thing if I need a sweetener. Why bother with artificial sweeteners when I know that a little bit of real sugar tastes good and is safe? I also have never been interested in using salt substitute. I find that it has a sharp, unpleasant aftertaste. And I don't see the point, since I eat a plant-based diet with few processed, high-sodium foods.

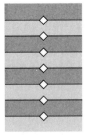

"Enjoying spices can make it much easier to eat a low-fat diet. Also, vinegar works well in place of salt in foods. Acids such as vinegar give you some salt punch. Have you ever tried hot-and-sour soup at a Chinese restaurant? It's the vinegar that gives it its kick."

—Robert Pritikin, director of the Pritikin Longevity Centers, in the book, *Shopping for Health: A Nutritionist's Aisle-By-Aisle Guide to Smart, Low-fat Choices at the Supermarket*

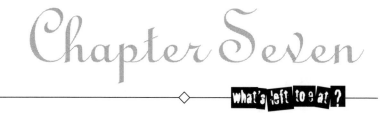

Chapter Seven

What's left to eat?

Summary: The Simple Truth

The truth is, the science of nutrition is complicated. The more we know about it, the more we realize how much we don't know. There are no easy answers, so don't let anyone fool you into thinking that they have it all figured out. If they don't acknowledge that there are a lot of "maybes," then they aren't being honest with you. What I'm telling you in this book is the best that anyone can know at the current time from a viewpoint that tries to remove the template of politics from the picture.

As I've said earlier, the science of nutrition is in its infancy. It's really only recently that the fuel we put into our bodies has been the center of so much interest. Even so, the number of dollars spent today on research about diet and nutrition is only a fraction of that spent on research about drugs and high-tech medical procedures.

That is certainly due, in part, to the fact that drugs are required to be tested before being approved for widespread use, as well as the fact that, in some instances, money is spent to test drugs in cases where it is unlikely that diet would have much impact, such as in the prevention or cure for AIDS.

However, politics is also undeniably part of the reason. No wonder. There's big money in drugs and high-tech medical interventions, just as there is big money to lose by some industry groups and their friends if there is a massive shift in eating habits. Like the tobacco industry, the dairy, egg, and meat industries are in a precarious position.

Consequently, we have a long way to go toward a good understanding of how the food we eat affects our health.

A Word About Bias

This newspaper is biased. Bias is not a deplorable state; rather it is a human condition. People are biased in all that they speak and write. The words or euphemisms that we use, the actions we choose to report on, and those we relegate to the "unnewsworthy" file are expressions of our bias. In this culture, the term "unbiased" is misused to mean the viewpoint of the majority.

The danger arises when the mainstream begins to label opposing viewpoints as being biased and thus somehow less accurate, academically incredible, and socially unacceptable. In this way, the unstated biases of the majority have the greatest influence on the readership. Since most Americans want to be in the know and part of a larger group, if not part of the mainstream, we tend to accept the majority's "unbiased" opinion as the truth, while ignoring those minority opinions labeled as "biased."

We feel that an openly stated viewpoint is a more equitable position to hold. It informs the reader that the human who is presenting this information has an outlook on the world which may color the presentation. This stand is an honest one, which is the most we may hope for.

—From *The Thistle*, an Alternative News Collective publication in Cambridge, Mass.

But we're getting there. We're moving ahead at warp speed. As a clearer picture comes into focus, it's quite apparent that the diet that is optimal for most of us is at odds with our traditions. The upside of this is that we now know that we have far more control over our own health than we had previously realized. Eat right and control other lifestyle factors, such as stress, exercise, and whether or not you smoke, and you can delay or prevent the onset of many diseases and conditions that were once thought to be the inevitable outcomes of old age or bad luck. The downside: Changing your eating habits can be a major-league challenge.

How challenging? Depends on your perspective. It also depends on the advice you get about what changes to make and how to make them.

The recommendations being given at this point by most mainstream health care providers and organizations are a mix of old-time traditions and current research. They straddle two worlds. "Choose two servings from the milk group each day," and "Choose lean meats and poultry," but at the same time, "Eat less fat, saturated fat, and cholesterol," and "Choose more fiber-rich foods."

The recommendations lack the clarity that most people need to put dietary guidelines into practice because they reflect the struggle taking place within a scientific and political community that has not yet come to terms with the fact that the science is not compatible with the tradition. Dietary recommendations are based not only on science but on value judgments, and those value judgments incorporate the desire to preserve traditions, as well as an assumption about what Americans will and will not change about their lifestyles.

Simple Keys to an Optimal Diet

The healthiest diet? That's the easy part. Remove the overlay of politics and cultural bias, and here you have it:

Eat a variety of foods. Make the bulk of the diet consist of whole-grain breads and cereal products, legumes such as beans and peas, vegetables, and fruits.

Get enough calories in your diet to meet your energy needs. Burn enough calories through regular physical activity to allow you to eat a reasonable volume of food, which, in turn, will help ensure that you will get all of the nutrients you need.

If you eat foods of animal origin, such as dairy products, eggs, and meat, make them no more than a side dish or minor ingredient in a dish. Animal products should be eaten as condiments rather than as a primary component in a meal. Most people would do best to weed these foods out of their diets, if not entirely, then considerably.

Limit the sweets and fatty, greasy, junk foods. Soft drinks and French fries are vegetarian, but they don't make for a nutritious diet. The more "empty calorie" foods you eat—foods that give you little nutrition for the calories—the more of the "good stuff" you displace or push off your plate. Most people can't afford to eat much junk without seriously compromising the nutritional quality of their diets.

Go easy on added fats in your diet, especially in the form of oils, margarine, butter, salad dressings, mayonnaise, fried foods, and fats that are added to foods in processing or preparation. Avoid them altogether if you can, particularly if weight control is an issue for you. A few nuts and seeds are fine if they are used as a garnish or very minor ingredient in a dish—a sprinkling here and there. This is especially true for children or people who are very physically active and need more calories. In these cases, added calories from plant sources of fat may be appropriate and desirable.

Choose foods as close to their natural state as possible. Processed foods are typically inferior to whole foods, since they have had fiber and nutrients removed or destroyed and often contain more sodium and other additives. Buy locally grown and organically grown produce when you have the choice.

If you feel uncertain about the nutritional adequacy of your diet or need individualized assistance, see a registered dietitian. I strongly advise you to find one that is familiar with plant-based or vegetarian diets. Call the American Dietetic Association's referral service (800-366-1655) to locate a vegetarian-friendly dietitian in your area. You can also call your health care provider, local vegetarian society, or community hospital for a referral. Also see Chapter 13 for more resources and Chapter 14 for a meal-planning guide.

Sound simple? That's the easy part. The real challenge is putting all of this into practice.

The Dietary Continuum

As you begin to change your diet, it may help to view the process as one that evolves over time.

When I made the switch to a plant-based diet as a teenager, I stopped eating meat overnight. But for years afterward, I ate cheese and eggs in much the same way that I used to eat meat—on sandwiches and as major ingredients in recipes. I ate cheese lasagna, macaroni and cheese, omelets, grilled cheese sandwiches, cheesy casseroles, and so on. These foods were a crutch until I figured out how to move on to the next step—replacing them with more foods of plant origin. My diet progressed in stages.

As my world expanded, I traveled more widely, made new friends, and ate in ethnic restaurants where I was exposed to cuisines of other cultures. Many of these foods contained little or no animal products. I tried my first Indian curries and Ethiopian lentils that I pinched with a piece of thin, spongy bread called injera and ate with my fingers. Chinese stir-fries were tame—I tried gluten dishes and miso soup for breakfast. Falafel sandwiches, couscous, and tabouille. Who knew the world of food was so vast and that people all over the globe could cook so well? My Midwestern peas-and-carrots upbringing became a distant memory.

The point is, you may find your diet moving along a continuum, from less to more foods of plant origin, as you gain familiarity and confidence and as your skills increase. Be aware of where you are in the evolution of your diet so that you don't become stuck in the "cheese and eggs rut" (see below).

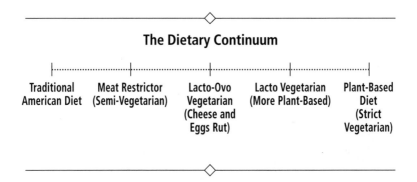

The Dietary Continuum

Traditional American Diet	Meat Restrictor (Semi-Vegetarian)	Lacto-Ovo Vegetarian (Cheese and Eggs Rut)	Lacto Vegetarian (More Plant-Based)	Plant-Based Diet (Strict Vegetarian)

Make Changes, Move At Your Own Pace

One school of thought says it's easier to make gradual changes in one's diet, and another says it's better to make big changes overnight. The idea is that any change is difficult, whether you are making big changes or little ones, and that by making bigger changes at the outset, you'll see the benefits faster and will find it easier to stick with the new program.

I take a point of view somewhere in between. In my practice, I have found that most people change their diets gradually. It's a practical matter. Unless you immerse yourself in the new lifestyle by attending a special retreat or moving in with someone who lives that way, learning by example and getting lots of support, it is virtually impossible to learn all of the new skills you need in order to switch overnight and be able to function the next day. Even if you took the "immersion" approach, you'd need to stay long enough to pick up the skills you would need to keep you going once you were out in the real world again.

I find that most people find a comfortable starting point and go from there. They learn and practice and muddle through at their own pace, making changes a step at a time.

On the other hand, I think it's important to be realistic about the starting point and your rate of progress. The "I'm cutting back on red meat" routine and "We're using more olive oil these days" just doesn't make it. If you're serious about making a change in lifestyle, then you'll need to make substantial changes today and be honest with yourself about your rate of progress.

But first, let's consider your starting point. If you are eating the typical American meat-based diet, then it may be wise to begin by simply cutting your meat portions in half and working on incorporating three or four meatless meals into your diet each week. But don't let this go on forever. Do this over a reasonable period of time—three or four months should do it.

Once you've mastered this step, go ahead and discontinue your use of meat, high-fat dairy products, and eggs. At the most, include them as condiments or minor ingredients in the dishes you eat. Eliminating animal products completely from your diet may not be necessary for optimal health, but many people find that the less of these foods they eat, the less they want them. They stop buying them altogether, and finally break out of the rut of giving these foods center stage.

Get the support you need to adapt to a vegetarian diet (see Chapter 13), and continue learning so you can refine your diet from there, making gradual changes from that point on. Be kind to yourself and don't expect perfection, it will take time to develop the skills and habits that will make this eating style second nature. Given time, though, it will happen. Part Two of this book will give you a good start.

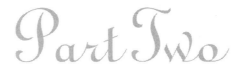

Getting from Here to There

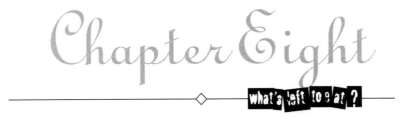

Chapter Eight

What's left to eat?

The Optimal Diet is Outside Our Culture

The dietary recommendations that we usually hear in the U.S. are ethnocentric. "Made in America." They come from the point of view that a meal is centered around a piece of meat, or that animal products—meat, eggs, or dairy—are central ingredients. They also assume that it's going to remain that way, that we want to hang on to our traditions.

The fact that the science is at odds with our traditions creates conflict. Eating healthfully, it seems, is incompatible with hot dogs and apple pie. The result is confusing, mixed messages about what we should and should not eat, cookbooks giving 1,001 ways to fix chicken and fish, and other ineffective programs and educational materials that fall short of the goal or miss the point entirely.

It's very important for you to recognize this if you are to successfully break out of the American diet mindset and make the transition to a healthier way of living. Being aware of the issue of culture will help you make sense

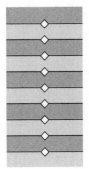

An American opinion poll conducted by The Wall Street Journal and published in June 1996 revealed that the No. 1 thing that Americans would do in a world without health consequences was to eat all the sweet, salty, high-fat foods they wanted. According to The Wall Street Journal:

"That was particularly true of women 18 to 34 years old, of whom 54% chose their low-fat diets as their biggest sacrifice to health. Although no other choices came close, No. 2 was having sex without taking safe-sex precautions."

of the conflicting messages that you may see and hear as well as maintain a realistic point of view concerning your goals.

You Are Here

If you were raised in North America or Western Europe, then your eating habits probably reflect the culture's meat-and-potato ways.

Imagine for a moment that your eating style and food preferences are just one dot on a map of diverse eating patterns from around the world. You are here, in the land of meat and potatoes, but around you, scattered around the map of the world, are rice and vegetable ways, beans and grains ways, pasta and vegetable ways, and many other styles of eating that may be foreign to you. You are probably unaware of these differences most of the time—secure in your own bubble of culture that perpetuates its unique customs and shields you, to a large extent, from the ways of others.

We are shielded in many ways from eating styles that are outside our culture. Chinese restaurants in the U.S. serve "Americanized" Chinese food, with large amounts of meat added, or special dishes created just to appeal to the American palate. Italian restaurants serve spaghetti sauce with ground meat mixed into the sauce or lasagna with ground meat added to the layers of what would traditionally be only pasta and cheese. It's the same story with Mexican foods. Large amounts of meat and gobs of cheese and sour cream are added to what would otherwise be healthful dishes made with tortillas, beans, and other vegetables.

We are surrounded by American-style restaurants, where a piece of meat that could serve four to six people is served to one. Vegetables are side dishes and are microscopic in size in comparison to the meat-based entree. Venture anywhere outside your home, and you'll find a fast-food restaurant on every corner serving hamburgers, fries, fried chicken, chicken nuggets, shakes, and fried apple pies.

Supermarkets stock American-style frozen entrees such as fried chicken and salisbury steak with gravy. Go to a friend's home for dinner or to a social occasion and you are likely to be met with a meat-and-potatoes meal. Buck the system, and you're likely to end up having the salad and a broccoli spear for dinner. Maybe a baked potato and a brown-and-serve roll, hold the butter.

This is our culture. Yes, it's changing. We are increasingly becoming a more sophisticated, multicultural community in which people from other ends of the earth are bringing new foods to our collective table. But we're a long way from the time when good-tasting, healthful food is readily available around the corner, down the street, or at your neighbor's house. It's going to take a lot more time before our customs change that significantly. In the meantime, know it and cope.

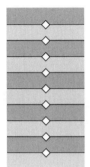

Did You Know...

In big cities, when I order Chinese food at a restaurant, I usually ask if they have any greens available. I order them as a side dish. Often, the restaurant orders Chinese greens to serve to its own staff, or it may save the leaves from snow pea pods to steam and serve to the staff. These greens are not actually offered on the menu, since Americans are not familiar with them and would be unlikely to order them. But they are delicious and super-nutritious.

Getting There: Seeing the Goal Realistically is the First Step

It bears repeating: The optimal diet is outside our culture. That fact by itself explains why most of us find it so difficult to change our eating habits. Even though we may know what is best for us and may honestly want to change, it's very difficult to pull it off.

Just realizing this fact is the first big step toward achieving your goals.

If you realize where the obstacles are to adopting a new and more healthful dietary tradition, then you can begin to work at getting around them or find other ways of coping. You will also be much more likely to spot the half-truths, distracters, and other pitfalls that line the path to your goal and confuse other, less savvy, folks. You will have your goals much more clearly in sight if you are aware of the ways in which culture, tradition, and the politics and economics of diet and nutrition affect the messages you hear from various sources. It pays to be an educated consumer.

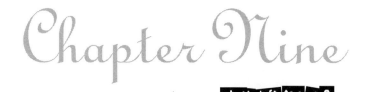

Making the Change At Home

Sometimes the easiest place to practice new skills is in your own backyard—or your kitchen, in this case. You have the most control over what you eat when you fix the food yourself. You have more choices when you are in your own home than in a restaurant or as a guest at someone else's house.

Think of your home as Command Central. It's your base, the place that you can count on for consistency in environment. You may never know where you'll travel to next or in which restaurant you'll find yourself, but at home, you can always count on the right foods being in your refrigerator and cupboards. At home, you can have a routine established that is supportive of and suitable to your lifestyle, whether you are a cook-it-from-scratch full-course meals type of person or someone who needs to grab something quick and be out the door.

It just takes planning. And practice. And a little know-how.

Are We in This Together?

First question: Are you going it alone, or is there a partner or family to consider? Are the others committed to making the change?

I was involved with a counseling case several years ago in which a couple raising a 2-year-old daughter were having a disagreement over diet and lifestyle that threatened their marriage. The man, an avowed meat and potatoes eater, wanted to take the little girl to McDonald's and to include meat in her diet at home. The woman, a health-conscious, strict vegetarian, wanted to raise the child on a low-fat vegetarian diet that excluded all foods of animal origin, including eggs and dairy products. There didn't seem to be any hope of compromise.

Although the child was still being breastfed, she was also eating table food and would soon be attending birthday parties at friends' homes and outings that might take her to fast-food restaurants and Chuck E Cheese. I was called to sit in on the couple's therapy sessions to provide expert advice and input on issues of diet—"just the facts, ma'am."

I followed this couple for three years, through the growth of the child and marital separation of the parents, through a custody battle, and through one or two reconciliations. There is actually no happy ending to report for this story. I lost contact with the couple when the woman had given in for the sake of family unity and had begun eating meat herself. I heard from her once more about a year later, and there had been yet another separation.

The story illustrates just how serious the matter of choice of diet can be in a family setting, or even within a couple. When everyone works together toward a common goal, the environment that is created can be especially supportive and strong. On the other hand, disparate lifestyle choices can be quite disruptive. If you are "going it alone," be aware of the potential stress that your alternative lifestyle may place on other relationships. Be prepared to discuss this with the significant people in your life and to work toward a plan for dealing with the issue in ways that are acceptable to all.

No Dictators Allowed

It's more convenient when everyone in a family agrees to eat the same way. Otherwise, the result can be having to prepare two different meals.

When I was a child, my mother announced one day at dinner that she had become a vegetarian and would no longer be eating meat. For the next several years, she prepared the usual meat-and-potatoes-one-vegetable-a-salad-and-bread meal for the rest of the family and ate either an omelette, or a cheese-and-pickle sandwich on whole-wheat toast herself. No variations. She fixed her own separate entree and ate what she could from the rest of the family's meal. Not another word was said about her

Can the Whole Family Eat This Way?

A low-fat plant-based diet can be appropriate for everyone, young and old alike. Most experts agree that while adults fare well on a diet that has 10 to 15% of its calories from fat, young children need more fat in their diets—at least 20% of calories—in order to get enough calories to meet their energy needs.

In families with small children, offering between-meal snacks is often a good idea and helps ensure that energy needs are met. Bean burritos or tacos, popcorn, bagels, a bowl of cereal, or a sandwich half are all good choices that children love.

Kids can generally tolerate some higher-fat foods that adults may wish to avoid. Since kids are growing and developing rapidly, and fat is a concentrated source of calories, adding a little peanut butter to an apple slice or a sliver of avocado on a sandwich won't hurt and can help boost a child's calorie intake. Plant foods are bulky, and little tummies fill up quickly, so the extra fat helps ensure that kids get the calories they need.

If you add some higher-fat foods to your child's diet, however, stick with plant sources of fat, rather than animal sources, which raise blood cholesterol levels. Peanut butter, almond butter, seeds (for older children who aren't as likely to choke) such as pumpkin, and seed butters such as tahini (used in bean dips), are good choices.

For more information about plant-based diets for children, refer to the resources listed in Chapter 13.

decision, and she went on eating this way for years.

Interestingly, over the next several years—and with not a word said about it—one by one, the kids in my family all went vegetarian as well, leaving my father the odd man out. Consequently, my mother began fixing less and less meat and instead began creating a wide range of more healthful, plant-based dishes, finally breaking out of the fatty cheese-and-eggs rut. We eventually arrived at the point where my mother would prepare a wonderful vegetarian meal for the entire family and would boil a hot dog for Dad. He began to rebel and showed his disapproval by first proclaiming that the meal had not been adequate, then getting up from the table and toasting a frozen waffle for himself. Those were stressful times.

Unlike my first story, this one ends on a positive note. Today, my parents are still married after nearly 50 years and are sharing wholesome, healthful, plant-based meals together. My father stopped resisting years ago, and my mother has perfected a wide range of delicious vegetarian dishes that everyone enjoys. Although my siblings and I are spread out across the country and no longer share daily meals together as a family, we all eat plant-based diets to this day.

The experience with lifestyle change that I had with my own family showed me that, first, it does cause a measure of discord when eating habits or food preferences are widely divergent within a family. My father didn't appreciate being served hot dogs for dinner, and when we kids finally joined our mother in eating a vegetarian diet, my father was upset. He thought that children needed meat to be healthy. Of course, since there was no discussion about the issue, nobody taught him that this was not the case.

Second, people do learn by example. I believe that, although she did-n't speak about it, my mother sent a powerful message to her children with her actions. Had she been preachy or tried to push everyone to follow her lead, we may well have resisted. People prefer to have the freedom to make their own choices.

As the years passed and I continued to eat a plant-based diet, others who are close to me have changed their eating habits—some adopting veg-etarian-style diets—without me having spoken a word about my own choices or prompting them to change theirs. I've merely set an example.

No Need to Be the Hall Monitor, Either

Here's a common scenario when I see a client for a private nutrition consultation: A woman makes an appointment with me to learn about the dietary changes that her husband needs to make for health rea-sons. Sometimes, a woman will call to make an appointment for the cou-ple to see me together for a problem that he has, and when the appoint-ment date arrives, she shows up alone.

The explanation: She's the one who does the cooking, so he decided he did-n't need to attend. This scenario could, of course, be played the other way around, with the husband attending for the wife, or any partner attending for another partner. But the first version is the one I commonly see. I've even had men attend sessions with their wives, only to act astonished when I direct a question to them, as if they were only innocent bystanders who happened, coincidentally, to be sitting in my office. "Don't ask me," they've said. "She does all the cooking."

"But you aren't always together, are you? What would you do if you were by yourself at a restaurant? What if you were together but at a big party and had to eat from a buffet line?"

"I don't know, but you need to talk to her."

It's a scene I've witnessed many times.

It's great when family members are supportive of other family members' lifestyle changes, and when everyone gets involved by learning and pitching in to make the transition easier. But I've also seen family members become frustrated when one or more don't care to take responsibility themselves for the changes that they need to make.

We each must take responsibility for our own choices. Understand that cajoling and trying to force another person to make a lifestyle change is rarely successful. You will, however, probably succeed in making yourself miserable and everyone resentful.

It bears repeating: The best way to help others make comprehensive lifestyle changes is to set a good example yourself. Teach by example. Your example may be more powerful than words. It may take months, or years, but others do notice.

I realized that when I looked back at all of the years that my mother silently ate her vegetarian meals. For years she ate her food and never said one thing to try to convince the rest of the family to change. But her consistency and resolve were hard to miss. She set an example that she may have thought had gone unnoticed, until one by one, each on his or her own terms, her children all followed suit. Even my father came around eventually, when he was good and ready.

Getting Junior to Eat His Vegetables

It's generally a losing battle to try to force people to do things they don't want to do, and kids are no exception. Before you lose any sleep over what Junior will and will not eat as you aim to bring the family around to a healthier way of living, here are some tips that may ease the transition:

Like everyone, children prefer a measure of freedom. They want to have choices. If your child turns his or her nose up at a meal, offer one or two substitutes for specific items. If your child still refuses, let it go. Your child won't starve, and the next meal will bring new choices.

Get your child involved in shopping for food. Children are more likely to eat what they have had a hand in choosing. If you are buying peaches from a bin, let your child pick out two or three. If you are buying boxed cereals, let your child decide between two choices. Older children can be given more responsibility. You could give an older child, for instance, the task of going to the other side of the store and finding a loaf of whole-grain bread or a couple cans of kidney beans for making bean chili.

Bring a spirit of adventure to trying new foods. At the supermarket, decide together to try something totally new. Experiment with jicama, or star fruit, or a mango or papaya. Show your child that it can be fun to try new things. If you find that you don't like something, that's okay, too. No harm done. When you take a chance with unfamiliar foods, some work and some don't. You may hit upon a few duds, but you'll probably find some new favorites, as well.

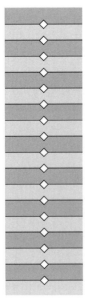

Dr. Antonia Demas of the Food Studies Institute has developed a program in which she goes into children's classrooms to teach them about food through a hands-on cooking demonstration. She exposes kids to foods from other cultures, then serves those same foods in the school cafeteria. Dr. Demas has found that children who are exposed in the classroom to new foods are 5 to 20 times more likely to choose those foods when they are offered in the cafeteria, as compared to children who were not previously exposed to the foods.

In a program for schools in Santa Fe, N.M., Dr. Demas helped children make couscous salad in teams. The children had 20 ingredients from which to choose, including three types of beans. Given the option of choosing which ingredients they would use, the kids used 17 out of the 20 ingredients. After preparing the salads and giving their "original recipes" names, the children discussed the food and voted for their favorite salad.

GOOD FOODS, BAD FOODS

Get your child involved in preparing meals. Children are more likely to eat what they have had a hand in preparing. Supervise young children and let them help with simple tasks such as retrieving items from the pantry or dumping prepared ingredients into a pot. Older children can help peel fruits and vegetables for salads or assemble ingredients for other dishes.

Plant a windowsill herb garden, grow a pot of tomatoes on the back porch, or cultivate a full-size vegetable garden in your backyard. Learning about foods by having the direct experience of raising them is fun and helps children develop an appreciation for their wholesomeness.

Set a good example yourself. Children can spot a broccoli-hater; don't think you can hide. If you turn up your nose at cooked kale or grimace at the mention of whole-wheat fettuccine, your child is likely to pick up on it and model the same behavior. Keep your opinions about food preferences to yourself unless they are positive ones. Let your child decide what he or she likes.

You don't have to eat something that you don't like, and you don't need to worry if your child doesn't like some foods, either. We all have food preferences. There are hundreds of different vegetables, fruits, and grains; if you don't like one or another, there are plenty of others to take its place.

Children often prefer different foods at different times. This week, a child may hate carrots, and next week mashed potatoes may be out. Or your child may want to eat nothing but bananas for a stretch of time. Don't worry about it. Food jags like these are usually temporary and are unimportant in the scheme of things.

Continue to set an example of good eating habits yourself and offer your child choices and substitutes when necessary. Take a "no big deal" attitude.

It's the Politics of Your (Child's) Plate

Children learn by example. Parents can model good eating habits at home, but what do children learn by meals served at school?

In the past few years, dramatic changes in the nation's school meals program have been initiated. These changes were sorely needed, as school meal regulations had not been substantially revised in 50 years, and a comprehensive study of school lunches showed that only one school in the country had meals that met the Dietary Guidelines for Americans. Almost without exception, school meals were found to be low in fiber and high in sodium, fat, saturated fat, and cholesterol, with nearly 40 percent of the calories in the meals coming from fat.

Complicating matters, the school meals system had been set up in a way that encouraged a high intake of fat- and cholesterol-laden foods. School meal regulations are under the jurisdiction of the U.S. Department of Agriculture. Schools receive government commodities, including beef, butter, and cheddar cheese, which are freely worked into menus to reduce costs. For 50 years, in order for schools to be eligible for federal reimbursements, meals had to follow a set pattern that required them to include a predetermined amount of meat and milk. A few meat substitutes were permitted to be used, but guidelines for using them made it an impractical alternative. Consequently, the system perpetuated an eating style that was at odds with today's Dietary Guidelines.

Under the first term of the Clinton Administration, sweeping changes in federal school meals regulations were proposed, including abolishing predetermined menu patterns and, instead, creating a system in which meals are evaluated on their overall nutritional composition. In other words, rather than requiring that a meal contain a set number of servings from individual food groups, any meal that could be shown to be nutritionally adequate (lunches would need to meet one-third of the Recommended Dietary Allowance for nutrients) would be acceptable. For the first time, the U.S.D.A. would also be required to conform to its own Dietary Guidelines in its school meals, and schools would have to show that they were reducing the fat, saturated fat, cholesterol, sugar, and sodium content of meals and boosting fiber.

The new system, Nutrient Standard Menu Planning, made it much easier for schools to incorporate ethnic foods and meatless entrees into menus—foods that tend to lower the fat, saturated fat, and cholesterol levels of menus and boost fiber. Increasing the flexibility of meal planning in this way promised not only to improve the nutritional profiles of school meals but to accommodate the food preferences of an increasingly multicultural student body, as well.

Currently, all schools have the option of using a nutrient-based menu planning system. The reality, however, is that most will not make use of it

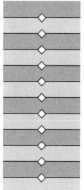

The next time you hear about a friend's low-fat diet, the next time you see a kitchen stocked with low-fat cookbooks and fat-free snacks, consider this: Three of the fastest-growing food categories in America are hamburgers, French fries, and chicken nuggets.

For the fourth year in a row, America is not eating more better-for-you foods, even as new low-fat items show up daily on supermarket shelves, according to a survey published this week by the NPD Group in Rosemont, Illinois.

—*The New York Times*, November 20, 1996,
in "Fattening of America: Less is No More"

in the near future. Throughout efforts to reform the school meals program, some groups had vested interests or stood to lose if schools abandoned the old "food component" system and instead adopted the new method of menu planning. Segments of the food industry, and some groups of school food service professionals, lobbied for a law that would supersede the U.S.D.A.'s ruling and permit schools to continue to use the old system. This law was passed along with legislation that significantly loosened procedures for ensuring that schools complied with mandates to meet the Dietary Guidelines.

Today, therefore, schools have the choice of using a nutrient-based system of menu planning or continuing to use the old system. Most schools plan to continue to use the old system. Although schools are required to demonstrate that they are making efforts to improve the nutritional quality of meals, compliance will be loosely monitored, and no punitive action can be taken if schools do not comply. You might say, then, that efforts to reform the nation's school meals program have been "two steps forward and one step back." At least it's a start.

Stocking Your Kitchen

A woman once hired me to come into her home and purge her cupboards and refrigerator of anything that didn't fit with the new lifestyle she had chosen. She wanted a clean, fresh start, and she didn't want to be tempted by junky snack foods and fatty meats and dairy products that were still lurking on the premises. After saving what we could, we dumped the rest into a big trash bag, then set out to the supermarket to restock her kitchen and fill in the gaps.

You don't have to go to such extremes yourself. It's okay to use up what you've got. Then, as you shop for fresh supplies, begin buying foods that fit with your new goals.

I like to keep a scrap of paper near my refrigerator, and as I notice that I'm running low on an item, I make a note of it. When I finally head to the supermarket, I take my list along. Shopping only from a list can help keep you from making impulsive decisions and buying foods that you'd really rather keep out of the house. Plus, without a list, I'm bound to forget what I needed. Having that list with me saves me from having to run back to the store for the garbanzo beans.

Some days, I shop strictly from the list and make a bee-line for only what I need. Other times, I walk up and down every aisle, taking the time to look at everything to notice what's new and try some new products. If I'm getting a little bored with my usual routine, I may even go to a different supermarket or a specialty food shop to look for something different and to get inspired.

What's Your Shopping Style?

People have different shopping styles, depending on their lifestyles and personalities. Some people plan menus for the week, then draw up corresponding shopping lists. This gives them a high degree of

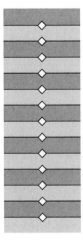

Try Ethnic for a Change of Pace

If you've never shopped at an ethnic grocery store, you might find it interesting. Most big cities—and even many small communities—have them. They can be Indian, Asian, Greek, Jewish, you name it. I never realized how many different kinds of lentils there were until I went with an Indian friend to her local Indian market where I saw red, yellow, black, brown, and orange ones. Indian music was playing in the store, and the aroma of Indian spices was everywhere. The store even sold small skillet-like pressure cookers from India for cooking dried beans and lentils. It was quite a unique environment and a nice change of pace. Check your phone book to see what's available in your area or ask friends and neighbors.

GOOD FOODS, BAD FOODS

control, which can be good for someone who needs the structure and is trying to establish a new routine.

Do what feels comfortable to you. What works for me is simply to have a variety of staples on hand in my cupboards and refrigerator, and to fix whatever I feel like having that day, depending on what's there and what I have time to make. My lifestyle is such that I may go out for dinner with a friend on the spur of the moment, or I might get tied up on a project or phone call and not eat dinner until late. Some days, I may feel like cooking something elaborate, and other days, I just grab something quick that I can heat and serve.

Despite my haphazard schedule, though, my eating habits are fairly disciplined. I eat well, even when it's a grab-and-go meal. I'll show you some easy, quick meal ideas in Chapters 14 through 16, as well as provide you with a meal-planning guide. Give yourself some time to develop these skills. It takes practice to learn how to make good choices and to eat well under varying conditions.

Cupboard, Fridge, and Freezer Staples

I like to buy foods that are versatile. When I have certain foods on hand, I know I'll always have something I can make for dinner. For instance, when I have canned beans in my cupboard, I have several options. I can use garbanzo beans to make my favorite bean dip, which also doubles as a sandwich filling. I can also rinse the beans and add them to a salad.

I can open a can of black beans, heat them in the microwave and eat them plain, with a little salsa on top, for a quick, nutritious meal. Or I can heat them in a skillet with some diced tomatoes, onions, and garlic, and serve that mixture over rice. I can even heat the beans, mash them (refried bean style), and use them to make black bean burritos, which I make using flour tortillas and adding chopped tomatoes, green onions, and salad greens. I may also take several kinds of beans and mix them together with other ingredients to make a many-bean chili.

So beans are versatile. Other versatile staples are rice and pasta. I usually keep several varieties of each on hand.

The following foods are good "starter staples" to put on your grocery list. For a detailed and extensive list of good choices and an in-depth discussion of supermarket shopping, see my book *Shopping for Health: An Aisle-by-Aisle Guide to Smart, Low-fat Choices at the Supermarket* (HarperPerennial, 1996).

---◇---

Starter Staples for Your Cupboard

Canned Goods

• Beans, canned or dry: baked vegetarian-style beans, black, kidney, garbanzo, pinto, navy, split peas, fat-free refried beans, and others
• Soups: lentil, black bean, split pea; natural foods brands may be lower in sodium than conventional brands
• Chili: vegetarian chili; as noted above, natural foods brands may be lower in sodium than conventional brands
• Bottled marinara sauce: you can dilute it with plain tomato sauce or crushed tomatoes if it's too rich-tasting straight from the jar

Dry Items

• Pasta: buy the kind made without egg yolks; try whole-wheat or part whole-wheat pastas
• Rice: basmati, jasmine, quick-cooking, arborio, long- or short-grain, quick-cooking; go for "brown" or whole-grain varieties
• Couscous: try whole-wheat couscous
• Whole-grain hot cereals: 7-grain, oatmeal, other grain mixtures
• Whole-grain cold cereals: shredded wheat, raisin bran, bran flakes, others
• Whole-grain pancake mix
• Pinto-bean flakes and black-bean flakes: I find these in natural foods stores; mix with boiling water and let set for five minutes for instant mashed beans
• Powdered egg replacer: usually found in natural foods stores; a blend of potato, arrowroot, and/or tapioca starch; very useful

Snacks

• Low-fat microwave popcorn
• Baked tortilla chips
• Low-fat, whole-grain crackers

Condiments

- Salsa: try different varieties—I've found pineapple, mango, raspberry, salsa verde, and others
- Flavored mustards: try raspberry, coarse-grained, honey-flavored, and others
- Fruit preserves: keep a variety on hand
- Chutney
- Vinegars: try mango, raspberry, seasoned rice, balsamic, herbed, or malt vinegar on potatoes
- Roasted red peppers: on sandwiches, or blend into garbanzo bean spread
- Natural, butter-flavored sprinkles
- Lite tofu and soymilks packaged in aseptic containers

Starter Staples for Your Refrigerator

- Fresh fruit (keep some in your fruit bowl): seasonal, buy locally grown and/or organic when possible; try mango, papaya with a squeeze of fresh lime, kiwi cups; keep several kinds on hand
- Fruit juice: calcium-fortified orange juice for those with an increased need for calcium, especially teens and young women
- Fresh vegetables: seasonal, buy locally grown and/or organic when possible; try superstars such as kale, broccoli, cauliflower, carrots, sweet potatoes, butternut, and acorn squash; be daring and experiment with some vegetables you've never before eaten—what's the worse that could happen?
- Breads (or keep in your bread box): whole-wheat pita pockets, whole-wheat flour tortillas (best refrigerated), bagels, coarse-grained whole grain breads and rolls

Starter Staples for Your Freezer

- Low-fat vegetarian burger patties
- Frozen juice bars and paletas
- Fruit sorbet
- Frozen soup vegetables and stir-fry mixes

Planning Ahead

Whatever the situation, planning ahead gives you the advantage of being in better control. If you are putting new eating habits into place, planning ahead can give you the extra support you may need at a time when your new skills are not firmly established. Put another way: planning ahead means being prepared.

At home, just having the right supplies on hand is the first step. We've already covered that one. The next step is to get a head start on your meals. You can do that in a number of ways. Some good ideas follow. You might also find it helpful to think about other ways to plan ahead that fit with your particular lifestyle or food preferences.

Getting a Head Start Can Be As Easy As:

Taking time to pre-wash and pre-cut fruits and vegetables after shopping. Take 20 or 30 minutes when you come home from the supermarket to organize and pre-prepare some of your produce. For instance, wash and cut up vegetables such as carrots, broccoli, and cauliflower florets, green onions, zucchini and yellow squash, green peppers—whatever you have. Store them in airtight containers or plastic bags in the refrigerator.

When you are ready to fix a meal, you'll be able to use these ingredients to make a quick salad, steam as a side dish, add to a stir-fry, saute as ingredients in an entree, or set out with salsa for a before-dinner appetizer.

Fresh berries such as blueberries and strawberries are ready to add to breakfast cereals, pancake batter, or cooked cereals, or to serve in a dish (or a fluted champagne glass!) for dessert. They only need rinsing before use (buy organic when you can). If you have fruit on hand that is likely to spoil before you will eat it, consider cutting it up and making a fruit salad. A scoop of fruit salad is good in hot cereal or on a mixed green salad, too.

Fix a big salad or two that you can eat for two or three days. Use seasonal fruits in different combinations. Chopped apples, pears, and figs taste good together, and blueberries with sliced peaches, or cantaloupe chunks with blueberries, are a striking combination. You can even add chunks of fruit— pears, apples, oranges—to a mixed green salad for a change of pace. One of my favorite green salads is baby spinach with sliced strawberry halves. Serve it with a low-fat poppyseed dressing or a splash of raspberry vinegar.

Other options: make a big, mixed green salad, a low-fat or fat-free vinai-grette coleslaw, tomato cucumber salad, marinated vegetable salad, four bean, or carrot, pineapple, and raisin salad.

When you make rice, make more than you need. Store leftover rice in the refrigerator, it can keep for a week or two if you store it in an airtight container. Leftover rice can be reheated in the microwave and served with steamed or stir-fried vegetables. Black beans, ratatouille, or bean chili are delicious served over rice. So is lentil soup — after heating, let it set for a few minutes to thicken first. You can serve leftover rice with bean burritos, and you can use it to make rice pudding. Add it to soups, stews, or jambalaya.

When you make such dishes as vegetable lasagna, casseroles, bean chili, and home-made soups, make enough to freeze some for another meal. You won't spend much extra time, if any, making a large batch, and you'll have a heat-and-serve meal on hand for a day when you don't have time to cook.

Do the same thing with muffins, whole-grain cookies, and quick breads. They freeze well, and you'll be so glad you did it. When you make pancake batter, you can make extra and store it in the refrigerator to use again later that same week. Just be sure to cover it tightly so it doesn't dry out.

Chapter Ten

◇ — What's left to eat?

Eating Out

Eating out happens to be one of my all-time favorite forms of entertainment. It's an aspect of traveling that I eagerly anticipate. At home, I enjoy experimenting with new restaurants as well as catching a quick meal at an old favorite. If the atmosphere is right, I can be temporarily transported to another city or another part of the world—a mini vacation in the middle of a harried work week.

Okay, I have a fertile imagination. But if I've just returned from a trip out of town, and my refrigerator is empty at home, I can grab a meal out and feel nurtured as well as nourished. Eating out is great fun, it's hassle-free (because I don't have to cook or clean up), and sometimes it's a time-saver. For many people, it's a way of life.

On the other hand, I also know people who avoid restaurants altogether. They only eat at home, where they can control the menu and monitor the food preparation. At home, they can be sure that no fat has been added to their food. At home, they aren't tempted by fat-laden entrees and rich desserts. They don't have to pick apart menus in search of healthy

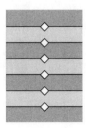
At the same time, America is big on restaurant junk food, feasting on almost eight million more orders of French fries, nearly six million more hamburgers, and five million more servings of chicken nuggets in a two-week period this year than last, the survey found.
—*The New York Times*, November 20, 1996, in "Fattening Of America: Less is No More"

options, and they don't have to explain their persnickety ways to their companions or apologize to the wait staff.

If the latter sounds like you, may I offer a piece of advice? Get out and enjoy yourself at restaurants, but go with an attitude of assertiveness and optimism. It is getting easier to find what you need at restaurants, and with a little coaching, you should be able to enjoy meals away from home with a minimum of fuss. It is possible, but it takes some practice and skills-building. I've got some great suggestions to share with you in this chapter.

You won't be alone. In fact, a 1992 survey conducted for the National Restaurant Association found that almost one out of five people—or about 20% of us—seek meatless entrees when we go out to eat. More low-fat and plant-based dishes are available now than ever before, and the number is going to continue to grow.

Restaurant Survival

Times are changing, but do remember that we live in a culture that caters to a "meat and potatoes" tradition. Is it any wonder that the majority of what we find on restaurant menus is heavy on the meat and dairy products—cheese, creamy sauces—and skimpy on the grains, vegetables, and fruits?

We live in the land of 16-ounce rib-eye steaks and 8-ounce pieces of fish. Restaurants serve a half of a chicken. These Flintstone-sized servings of meat are generally teamed with vegetable and grain side dishes that are dwarfed in comparison. Relegated to the side of the plate, the message is that these foods are of lesser importance. Fruits play an even smaller role—they're usually the garnish; a twist of orange or a sliver of melon teetering on the edge of the plate.

Restaurant food also tends to be cooked with a great deal of fat. Foods are fried, and chefs use a heavy hand when it comes to adding salad dressings. Butter and oil are typically used freely.

These are the realities, but they are limitations that can be overcome. For instance, I usually eat out only at restaurants that I know are going to have several healthful menu options from which I can choose. I don't even bother with some of the chain stores that balk at making a dish "my way" or don't have enough flexibility to make food to order. If I'm going out to eat with a group of people, I suggest a few restaurants that I know will offer several good choices and try to steer the group away from those that are more limited.

Here are some other tips I've grown to rely on over the years:

If pasta is listed on a restaurant menu, I'm all set. Even if the toppings sound disastrous—Alfredo sauce, "creamy tomato dressing"—I don't give up. I love any interesting form of pasta—a fresh linguine or fettuccine, or multicolored rotini—tossed with steamed, fresh vegetables, fresh herbs, and just a touch of olive oil. It doesn't matter that this isn't listed on the menu. If the restaurant has pasta and vegetables, then I know that the chef can nearly always make a simple pasta primavera.

If baked potatoes are served as a side dish, I frequently order one as an entree along with two or three other vegetable side dishes or a salad. Often, the baked potatoes are huge and filling—my companions eating the steak usually admit that the potato and side orders or salad bar would have been enough. I may add some chopped broccoli and mushrooms to my potato, some salsa, black pepper, or maybe a sprinkling of Parmesan cheese for flavor.

At better restaurants, I scan the menu and look at the side dishes that are served with the various entrees. Many people don't notice them, but I zero right in. If you start with the mindset that a meal does not have to have a focal point or entree, then you open up options.

There are times when there are so many fabulous-sounding side dishes—and appetizers—on the menu that I have all I can do to narrow the selection down to three or four. I've had some wonderful meals that consisted of vegetable, fruit, and grain side dishes, a salad, and some terrific bread. Many times, I've wondered how anyone could have had room for the entree and what I would have missed if I had ordered one.

When a sandwich is listed on a menu as being served with potato chips or French fries, I take a look at the list of side dishes offered. I may ask to substitute a bowl of fruit salad, a baked potato, or a small green salad instead. If there is an additional charge, that's fine.

I go for atmosphere. If a restaurant has a particularly appealing atmosphere, or the view is spectacular, then I don't mind as much if my menu choices are more limited. There are times when it is simply difficult to find a worthwhile item on a menu, and when that happens, I don't fret too much if I can enjoy my surroundings. I can appreciate an ordinary tossed salad with crackers or a more-or-less mundane steamed vegetable plate with rice if I can listen to good music or bask in a spectacular view.

I don't even bother stopping at restaurants that serve poor quality, mass-produced food served in a noisy, chaotic atmosphere. Not only are my choices likely to be limited, but I know that the surroundings are not going to be pleasurable. I have several chain restaurants in mind when I say this. At one, the server once brought the dessert tray to the table, and it held plastic replicas of each of the desserts offered.

Instead, I seek out restaurants known for their attention to good service and fine-quality food, independently owned and run eateries, and ethnic restaurants. I'm more likely to find an interesting atmosphere, better-quality food, and more personal attention.

Restaurant Survival: Best-Kept Secrets and Helpful Hints

I've shared a few of the tips that work for me when I eat out. But the best people to ask for advice about eating in restaurants are the real experts: restaurant owners and chefs themselves. They are the ones who know what goes on behind the scenes and what customers can and can't get away with when they eat out.

When I asked some of these experts for advice about how to get healthful, good-tasting food at restaurants, I got an enthusiastic response. Most had some very helpful tips to share, although you'll also notice that a couple of the responses indicated a less-than-full understanding of what "healthy-fare customers" are looking for. Since that is part of the reality of restaurant-dining, I've printed their responses here in their entirety. Also, a few of the respondents gave similar suggestions. I've printed those responses, too, because I think that they emphasize some key points.

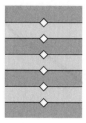 For additional, specific suggestions for ordering meals at various types of restaurants (Italian, Mexican, Chinese, and so on), you might want to refer to my first book, *Simple, Lowfat & Vegetarian* (Vegetarian Resource Group, 1994). It includes lists of great choices, dishes to avoid, and sample menu makeovers. Some additional tips for restaurant choices are given in Chapter 12.

GOOD FOODS, BAD FOODS

Here's What the Experts Want You To Know...

"Unfortunately, when people go out to restaurants and ask for a healthful, plant-based alternative meal, many restaurants serve meals that are not well thought out. For example, they may just offer an ordinary pasta dish. How much the restaurant is willing to accommodate the needs of the guest depends upon its level of enlightenment or hospitality.

"One thing people can do is to go through the menu and take a look at all of the main courses. Look at the items that accompany the entrees. People can often put something together that suits them from those items.

"If you are out of town, you might want to stop at the local farmers' market. Find out whom they sell to—restaurants or only pedestrian traffic? If they sell to a restaurant, that restaurant may be a good bet for finding a healthful meal.

"Often it won't say this on the menu, but if you are concerned about fat, ask how a food is prepared. You may want to request that the item be prepared with olive oil or just steamed instead.

"One more point: when people ask for low-fat foods, some chefs interpret that to mean "not seasoned." You can end up with something bland and tasteless. Ask the kitchen to season your food but not to use fat, if that is what you are trying to avoid. Herbs, spices, and flavorful broths can add excitement without fat."

—Michael Romano, Executive Chef/Partner
Union Square Cafe
New York, N.Y.

"Better-class restaurants are likely to be more receptive to special requests from customers. Their patrons tend to be better-educated and more sophisticated travelers who are aware of health trends and are more likely to request healthful cuisine on a regular basis. Family chains such as Red Lobster, Olive Garden, Bennigan's, and Houilihan's are not as likely to be receptive or able to accommodate these special requests. Generally, their clientele are not as likely to demand it nor are they as likely to know what to ask.

"Keep in mind that a restaurant needs time to prepare a special meal, and chain-type restaurants are not as well-equipped to spend extra time on special requests. If you want vegetable- and grain-based cuisine, you need to call ahead. Ask the restaurant what it can provide you with in the way of this type of cuisine. A quinoa/garbanzo bean filet? You should also have a little idea of what you want, as well, so that you can offer some ideas yourself.

"If you want a non-meat meal and you are eating at a chain restaurant, ask what type of stock they use in cooking; it may be chicken or beef. If there is a particular ingredient, such as fat or meat, that you want to avoid, you might say that you are "allergic" to that item. The chef and manager will be all nervous—they'll be shaking in their shoes because they don't want to lose you as a customer—and you'll be more likely to get a dish without those ingredients!"

—Mark Dowling, Chef/Instructor
The Disney Institute
Orlando, Fla.

"Communication is the key to accommodating a guest in the best possible manner. The guest must simply tell the server what specific needs must be met. It is best if the kitchen isn't forced to have to second-guess the diner. For example, instead of asking for a vegetable plate, explain that you are on a diet … or you are a vegetarian … or maybe just not that hungry. If the kitchen knows what the guest desires, it they can suggest other possible solutions to satisfy him or her."

—Robert Del Grande, Chef/Partner
Cafe Annie
Houston, Texas

"Get a menu ahead of time so you're prepared with questions. Restaurants can usually fax a menu.

"Whenever possible, call the restaurant ahead and share your dietary concerns.

"If it's appropriate, ask to speak to the chef and ask her or him for recommendations.

"If a restaurant offers no vegetarian options, it will usually put something together for a customer. The more time there is to prepare, the better.

"At the restaurant, let your server know immediately that you'd like to have your food cooked with as little salt and fat as possible.

"When asking for substitutions, be specific. For example, if creamed spinach is the vegetable, and you'd like to avoid the cream, tell the server. Ask for simple wilted spinach instead, or something else that is available in the restaurant. The more information the kitchen and server have, the better.

"Be prepared to be surprised. Remember that the restaurant has prepared a menu that works for the system, and most of the people in the restaurant are ordering straight from the menu. Having a system is what makes it possible for the restaurant to run smoothly. Your request interrupts the system and it may not be possible for the kitchen to produce exactly what you want. Be flexible.

"Appetizers tend to have a higher vegetable/grain content and a lower fish/meat content.

"If you see an appetizer that appeals to you that you'd like to have as an entree, ask for a double order. Do something different—order three appetizers rather than an appetizer and an entree.

"Be prepared to pay for your request."

—Jody Adams, Chef
Rialto
Cambridge, Mass.

"It is a challenge to eat healthful meals in restaurants, but far less of one than it used to be! Restaurants like ours are shopping locally and seasonally and putting grains and vegetables at the center of the plate.

"When you read a restaurant menu and you're really hungry, it's very tempting to start with fettuccine with cream sauce, ravioli, or truffle-studded mashed potatoes. Instead, try a salad or cold appetizer. They may not sound as decadent or 'special-occasion-like' but can be delicious and inspired, and can remind you of how perfect fresh vegetables are. Instead of thinking of these items as less exciting, think of them as a way to measure the restaurant's ability to handle simple things well."

—Susan Feniger and Mary Sue Milliken, Owners
Border Grill
Santa Monica, Calif.

"I try to balance all my dishes with a different starch and vegetable. Often I use leafy greens such as kale, mustard greens, rapini, and so on, and locally grown produce whenever possible. As a result, my customers are assured of having at least 8 to 10 different vegetable choices available for substitutions according to their dietary needs.

"My advice would be first, to choose a restaurant with some variety in the vegetables and starches offered. Second, ask how they are cooked, since the wait staff will not always tell you up front. How much and what kind of fat is used? Do they season their vegetables? With what? Third, have mercy. Don't go overboard. You should enjoy eating out. Making it easier on the kitchen staff, especially on the first visit, will allow them to serve you better. A little olive oil or vinaigrette on the side will tell the kitchen that you care about the flavor of the food you eat, not just the nutritive value."

—Stewart Scruggs, Executive Chef
Zoot
Austin, Texas

"Perhaps the most obvious is that most restaurants are delighted to make a plate of their vegetable 'sides' available to guests on short notice. We can combine appropriate starches and vegetables and add a beurre blanc or other non-meat based sauce that may be on the line that night [author's note: pass on the beurre blanc—it's butter-based].

"Also, I would always be glad to make up a plate of some fabulous vegetable that is very fresh and seasonal if the guest is willing for the preparation to be very simple, such as baby carrots steamed, with fresh snipped herbs or wild mushrooms sauteed in butter [author's note: fat-free with some fresh lemon juice or with a touch of olive oil would be a better choice than butter!].

"The thing that is very difficult is the last-minute request (when the table has already been seated and we are in the middle of a rush) when that request is more complicated than what I previously described. I also can say that last-minute vegan requests can be very difficult to fill.

"On the final note, the best thing a guest can do is trust the kitchen to come up with a simple, fresh, satisfying plate. The less the customer insists on controlling, the better we can make it happen."

—Odessa Piper, Executive Chef and Proprietor
L'Etoile
Madison, Wisc.

"If a customer lives in an area that doesn't offer a 'greener' cuisine, plant-based choices are sometimes available in ethnic-type restaurants. Most 'non-American' cuisines are naturally more plant-based. In those types of restaurants, I may piece together my meal from the side order selections. Grains, vegetables, and condiments are usually available and sometimes

GOOD FOODS, BAD FOODS

prove more interesting than the entrees.

"Another thing to do is to choose smaller proprietor-operated establishments where you'll get more personal service. If the owner is seating you or cooking your meal, he or she is more likely to be open to your requests. By voicing your needs and making choices about how you spend your money, you can affect a change and gradually help bring food service to cleaner, greener, and healthier food choices."

—Burniece Rott, Executive Chef
Nature's Fresh Northwest
Portland, Ore.

"When eating out, be willing to accept some chicken stock. Many chefs use stocks liberally. Most of this use is prior to meal service. For example, rice is cooked with chicken stock in the morning, then reheated. By demanding absolutely vegan ingredients, you limit what the chef can do. Instead, just request 'something vegetarian.' [Author's note: chicken stock can be fatty, and chicken fat is not what you want. Request fat-free or cooked with a touch of olive oil instead. If it's cooked with chicken stock, I'd avoid it.] Aloha!"

—Peter Merriman, Owner
Merriman's Restaurant
Waimea, Hawaii

"First, don't be afraid to ask for what you want. In the restaurant business, service to the customer is of utmost priority, or restaurants will have no business. A server works for TIPS, which stands for To Insure Proper Service. Ask your server for help deciding what to order or ask what the chef would suggest. Try to stay away from chain establishments as much as possible. Be picky about your food choices. If customers everywhere tell chefs what they want, they'll eventually get it.

"Those of us involved in the Chefs Collaborative 2000 [author's note: a national network of chefs devoted to advancing sustainable food choices] want customers to become more aware and conscious of their daily food choices. We, as a collective group of chefs, will give the customer what you want. Portobello mushroom is an example of a vegetable that, when marinated and grilled, can be ordered as a meat substitute. An educated chef will have a major role in the development of this trend towards health and diversification away from processed food to fresh.

"As Chefs Collaborative 2000 grows around the country, we hope restaurant customers will notice the importance of chefs being involved in this organization and choose eating establishments where the chefs are involved in the collaborative."

—Gary Sloss, Executive Chef
The Forest Country Club
Ft. Myers, Fla.

"Most upscale restaurants do have a vegetarian choice on their menu, but one could order the vegetables from two different entrees to make one entree. Otherwise, calling the restaurant ahead and making a vegetarian request is always a good idea.

"(Vegetarian entree example from menu): BLACKEYED PEA AND WILD RICE PATTY with fire-roasted peppers, onion, squash, and mushrooms; served with bell pepper sauce."

—Elizabeth Terry, Owner
Elizabeth on 37th
Savannah, Ga.

"Ask for sauces on the side.

"Don't be afraid to request your favorite starch as a substitute for the daily selection.

"If the server does not respond to your request, politely ask to see the floor supervisor.

"Request a nutritional data chart on designated health cuisine items for more thorough profiles.

"Ask for a larger portion of vegetables.

"Call ahead of your dinner out to speak with the chef regarding desired food preparation."

—Tom Maier,
President, Agri-Culinary Enterprises and Chef, Cavanaugh's
Kalispell, Mont.

"The center of the plate is beginning to change. There has been a trend here in Boston of restaurant chefs using products straight from the farm. We have all become more responsible.

"Some advice to consumers from a chef's point of view:

"Seek out good restaurants where the chef has a decent reputation. This doesn't necessarily mean expensive. Avoid big chains and places of great volume. They shop for quantity, not quality.

"Talk to the waiter or waitress, being sensitive not to make too many requests, especially on a Friday or Saturday night. The objective of any good restaurant is to make sure the customer has the best experience possible.

"Seek restaurants that follow certain cuisine related to this particular diet. For example, Mediterranean or Asian. Don't go out to a fondue restaurant.

"A lot of chefs have meatless dishes on their menus but don't identify them as being 'vegetarian.' This is why it is important to talk to the server. Chefs have a problem with salt and fat. Simply ask for low salt/fat.

"In the past, I've had many customers call ahead of time to tell me of any special dietary restrictions. I would make a bowl of steamed fresh vegetables with plain couscous for a woman at least once a week. She would make a reservation and tell the person to inform me. This way, I had time to prepare the special couscous before service for it not to be a problem later during the dinner frenzy. Special requests should be well-communicated."

—Ana Sortun, Chef
Casablanca
Cambridge, Mass.

"Tell your server up front about your dietary needs, restrictions, wants, hopes, dreams…

Before you order, ask about oil, cream, butter—things that might be used in food preparation but may not be listed on the menu.

"Ask about the flexibility of the kitchen as far as creating new things or changing items on the menu. Don't assume anything is possible, but with the right attitude, you can usually get what you want.

"Ask about price increases (or decreases) for changes.

"Always act grateful for the special attention you are given.

"Call ahead if you feel the needs of your party are restrictive to see if this is the right restaurant for you.

"Rosie (one of our chefs) suggests being aware of menu catch-phrases: crispy means fried; au gratin means with cheese; scalloped means with cream; sauteed means cooked with oil or butter; creamy means the actual use of cream or eggs.

"All of these usually mean a higher fat content. She suggests looking for 'baked, broiled, roasted, or blackened' instead.

"Be sure to ask about hidden meats such as in a soup or sauce. They're not always listed but are quite often used."

—Theresa Girault, Owner
Carpe Diem
Charlotte, N.C.

"Here are a few tips on eating out; it can be difficult at times, I agree:

"Baked potatoes are often available—even in out-of-the-way places. Once, while traveling, I was thrilled to get a microwaved baked potato for dinner at a diner in southern New Mexico.

"Simple and pretty obvious: salad with dressing on the side, lemon, if available, or any fresh vegetable that can be steamed or briefly microwaved.

"If you are not strictly vegetarian, ask if a smaller portion of meat or fish is available. We offer both a large and a small portion of fish with steamed rice or potato and steamed vegetables.

"In some areas, it is most practical to take simple meals with you. Think in terms of camping. Oatmeal or other hot cereal is very easy to prepare (instant versions may be available in restaurants)."

—Lynn Walters, Chef and Owner
Natural Cafe
Santa Fe, N.M.

"I design my menu to have one vegetarian appetizer, made with portobello mushrooms, and one vegetarian entree, which is cappellini with vegetables, since we have so many vegetarians in Austin. If you want the most healthful meals, look for dishes with vegetable-based sauces, such as a yellow-pepper sauce, rather than dishes made with chicken or beef stock or cream, which are rich in fat.

"Vegetables that are steamed or sauteed with lemon juice are the most nutritious. Almost any vegetable tastes great if it's marinated in lemon juice or sherry vinegar before cooking. In our restaurant, vegetarians can also order a 'starch' plate, and they can choose from an assortment of starchy vegetables or grains such as mashed potatoes, potatoes cooked in vinegar, polenta, sweet potatoes, potato tarts, and others.

"Most people choose a particular restaurant for a reason; they want steak, or chicken, and so on. So, if you want to eat healthfully, you should go to a restaurant where you know you'll have several good choices. Call in advance and ask for something special. This is a service industry, and, as a chef, I'm happy to do it. Never be afraid to ask for what you want. That's how food trends in restaurants start. The restaurants that people call 'trendy' are those that listen to customers' needs. The way I look at it, if I have the ingredients that a customer wants in a dish, I'll make it. After all, it's a sale, and I think it's important to respond to customers' needs.

"As a chef, I need to hear about my customers' wants and needs in order to advance in my craft. But there needs to be consideration on both sides. Call ahead. Don't go at the busiest time and ask for something special without giving some advance notice. As a customer, if there are problems with the food service at a restaurant, approach the chef or owner with a solution, or suggestion for how it might be improved."

—David Garrido, Executive Chef
Jeffrey's
Austin, Texas

"1. Call ahead when making your reservations, and let them know that you have a special request. This gives restaurants a chance to plan ahead.

"2. Be considerate of your request, especially when the restaurant is busy."

—Caprial Pence, Owner
Caprial's Bistro & Wine
Portland, Ore.

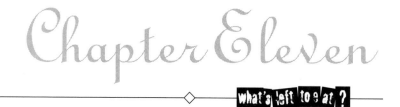

Chapter Eleven

The Social Side

You might have anticipated that changing your eating style would have presented certain challenges when you went out to eat at a restaurant, when you were traveling, or when you were faced with "what will I make for dinner tonight?" at home. But what you might not have expected is how a change in your eating style can affect relationships outside of your home, with extended family and friends.

Anyone who has tried to follow a weight-loss diet probably knows exactly what I mean. Announce to your host—especially if it's a family member or close friend—that you'd rather pass on dessert because you are trying to lose weight, and you are likely to have to dodge the ol', "Oh, come on. It's the holidays. You can have one piece," or duck the ever-popular, "But these are your favorite; I made them especially for you."

It can be very difficult for others to cope with the behavior of another person when that person chooses to behave in a way that is outside the cultural (or familial) norm. If your group of friends has enjoyed eating pepperoni pizza and swigging a few beers together every Friday night for years, and you decide that you are switching to the Veg-O-Matic, hold the cheese, with flavored seltzer water, it's bound to disappoint some people. It might be hard for them to put their fingers on exactly why things don't seem like as much fun anymore, but chances are good that the problem would be traced to your new-found healthy eating habits.

By choosing to follow a different dietary path, you are breaking with tradition. That can be especially hard within families. I remember when someone close to me changed his eating habits and stopped eating meat. His family traditions were heavily centered around food, and holidays and special occasions usually meant that his Italian mother and grandparents spent days or even weeks getting ready, preparing lots of family favorites. Entrees included meat of some sort, and even pasta dishes and sauces were cooked with Italian sausage and other meats.

His choice to forgo the foods containing meat created a great deal of friction within his family. The disapproval, sadness, and hurt were palpable. These foods represented love and tradition (maybe a little control, too), and it was unacceptable for him to reject them. He was straying from the clan, and the clan felt a strong need to pull him back into the fold.

The tug-of-war went on for years. Two low points included an attempt to trick him into eating meat that was present in a seemingly meatless dish, as well as his mother waving a piece of raw meat under his nose. She: "Mmmm. Doesn't this look good?" He: "No!"

After years of subtle and not-so-subtle pressure to get him to eat the food, time finally eased the tension. He didn't succumb to the pressure, so his mother began making a separate batch of food just for him—ravioli or another pasta dish made with a marinara sauce and no meat. Guess what? It became a new tradition.

Of course, there aren't always heavy emotional consequences associated with a person's change of eating style. Sometimes, the problem can be that it's just plain inconvenient for others when your eating habits are different than everyone else's. You have plans to go to someone's house for dinner, and they only know how to cook one thing: fried chicken, potato salad, gelatin mold salad, and biscuits. That's their "we're having company meal," and if you won't eat the food, you are really throwing a wrench into the works.

These are examples of the kinds of real-life experiences that many people find they must cope with when they make big changes in their style of eating. What are some effective ways of dealing with them?

Strategies for Success

Ultimately, your success in coping with social situations related to your diet will depend on your ability to develop some specialized skills. A positive attitude and a good sense of humor are a big help, too. The following tips will help to get you started:

1. Anticipate complications. Think through a potential tough spot and formulate an idea about how you might handle it. Do this before you find yourself in the thick of it.

For example, if your get-together with friends each week includes a mandatory rich dessert that you would prefer to avoid, you might decide to head off the problem in any number of ways. You might put yourself in charge of dessert this week and bring a gorgeous arrangement of tropical fruits accompanied by some low-fat cookies or an icy fruit sorbet. On another occasion, you might have a snack before you head out for the evening, so that you'll really mean it when you say, "I couldn't eat another thing."

2. Educate and inform others about your dietary needs. In some cases, it may really pay to explain to the people close to you just how serious you are about making changes in your eating habits. You might ask them up front for their support. You might tell them that you understand that your choice puts a measure of stress on some relationships. By being candid about your concerns, you may help others become aware of the impact that their own attitudes and needs may have on your ability to be successful in your efforts to eat well.

Not all dietary changes create stress within families. In my own family, the vices have always been desserts and coffee. Most of my relatives are the kings and queens of coffee-drinking. Dinner at the home of my parents is usually accompanied by coffee, followed by dessert and more coffee after the meal, dessert again later, and coffee throughout the evening. It's easy to succumb; if you do, you're up all night.

However, when I've mentioned that I'd prefer not to drink coffee, my mother has graciously set my place at the table with a water glass instead of a coffee cup and only offered coffee ("just asking to be sure") once. Likewise, when she announced her intention to decaffeinate herself, I no longer offered coffee to her when she came to my house. If she wanted some, she would have asked.

Over the years, some of my former clients have shared their favorite tips with me. Two stand out for times when the soft, sincere approach described above doesn't work. One person told me that he tells friends that he's "allergic to fat" and that he will become very ill if he eats fatty foods. He says that this works at restaurants, too, when he is explaining to the waiter that he wants his food cooked with no added fat.

In a similar vein, other clients have told me that the "blame it on a third party" approach is also effective, especially when the third party is a medical professional. They tell friends, family members, and business associates, "My doctor has strictly forbidden me to eat greasy foods." Works like a charm, they say.

3. Use the broken record technique—it works. It works. It works. Develop the ability to say no gracefully—over and over again, if necessary. When someone presses you to eat something that you don't wish to have, smile and say, "No, thanks." If they ask again, reply once more (with a smile and a shake of the head), "No, really, none for me." Again? "No, thank you."

One "no" might be enough for some folks, but others will hang in there for two or three. Eventually, they'll give up and leave you alone. Let people learn that when you say no, you mean it. Once you've set that expectation, people will be less likely to badger you. It will get easier each time you practice this assertiveness technique.

4. Be assertive. It's okay. It's okay to let your needs be known. There's no need to be shy about it. You can do it politely. This goes for times when you are with family and friends, as well as at other social and business functions, when you may need to ask for what you want at a restaurant or banquet.

I know someone who once ate very well at home but balked at asking for healthier fare when he attended business luncheons. His business associates were very traditional and conservative, and he didn't want to draw attention to himself and be branded as "different." This was the time of "real men don't eat quiche." Real men ate steak and potatoes, of course.

That was then, however. Ask him today how he handles it, and you'll hear a different story. He realized over time that attitudes had changed. These days, it's more likely that positive traits would be attributed to someone who obviously cares enough about his or her health to choose foods wisely. It looks good if you show that you care about your own health and fitness. Who knows? It may even lead to a promotion!

If you are a guest at a banquet, wedding, or other catered event, it's quite appropriate to ask for a special meal. You can call the hotel, country club, or restaurant yourself and make the arrangements directly, or you can ask the host or another representative to do so for you.

5. Don't preach. Trust me. You'll make a much better impression if you do your own thing and let other people eat what they want to eat in peace. There's no faster way to repel others than to nag them about their eating habits or to harass them with unwelcome lessons in nutrition.

I offer this advice as a nutritionist who happens to practice what she teaches, but does it quietly. I can tell you countless stories about the most unlikely people who have sought me out for advice about how to change their eating habits and have told me that they were able to approach me specifically because I didn't preach.

Realize that not everyone may be as motivated as you are to change their eating habits. I happen to believe that taking charge of one's health is a socially responsible thing to do, but I also know that trying to force people to change rarely works. As I've suggested earlier in this book, I feel the best approach is to influence others by setting a good example yourself.

6. Orient social events to activities rather than food. Let's face it. Most of us can eat anything once in a while—however rich, greasy, cholesterol-laden, and fiberless—and live to tell about it. It's what you do consistently that counts. But that's the catch. Consistency. If "once in a while" is daily— maybe even weekly for some people—that may be too often.

If you face social situations with friends, family, or business associates regularly, and they pose difficulties due to the type of food being served, you may want to consider making the occasions more centered on activities rather than food. This may not work in all instances, but it may work in some.

For example, if you get together with a particular friend each week to catch up over coffee and dessert, you might consider taking a walk together instead. Walk your dogs together. Go for an evening or morning stroll together. The chances are good that your friend would welcome the opportunity for a little extra exercise, too. You might ride bikes for a change of pace, or meet at the pool, depending upon the season.

Your Place or Mine?
Being a Gracious Host or Guest

You Are the Guest. Here is the scenario: you've been invited to someone's home for dinner, and you are wondering whether you should broach the subject of the menu. Of course, we're using common sense here. If you are invited to someone else's home for dinner once in a blue moon, then it probably won't make a great deal of difference if you eat a small amount of whatever fat-laden dishes they serve you. On the other hand, let's say that you do eat away from home fairly often, and you know that consistency counts. Should you tell your host of your food preferences? If you eat a plant-based diet, should you tell your host that you are a vegetarian?

As is often the case, there is more than one way to look at this issue, and more than one path you might choose. Here's what I suggest:

Size up the situation first. If this is someone with whom you are familiar, and if you feel comfortable in doing so, then I see nothing wrong with informing your host of your food preferences.

You can say it in a diplomatic, caring way, "Pam, I'm so looking forward to seeing you Thursday night, but I wanted to ask you about something. I've been trying really hard to eat a low-fat, high-fiber diet, and I'm trying to be consistent when I'm away from home. Can you give me an idea of what you are thinking of serving?"

From there, you can determine whether you'll have a problem. In being up front with your host, you will also give him or her an opportunity to change the menu to suit you. The host, for instance, might have been deciding between black bean soup as a starter with vegetable paella and saffron rice as the entree, and lamb shish kabobs with rice and pita pockets. Given your input, she may choose to go with the bean soup and paella.

On the other hand, let's say the host had decided on the shish-kabob dinner. Given your input, the host now has an opportunity to plan ahead and make your shish kabob with tempeh (a soy product) instead of meat, or simply to make more of the side dishes—extra vegetables, rice, and bread.

Another option you might consider—particularly if the host seems awkward or lacking in confidence that he or she can accommodate you—is offering to bring a dish of your own. You could bring enough so that others could try it as well. You might ask what the host is planning for the menu and bring something compatible.

For instance, if this is a summertime cookout featuring hamburgers, potato salad, and corn on the cob, you might offer to bring some meatless burger patties to grill. If the host is planning to make grilled steaks, you could offer to bring a delicious grain- and vegetable-based casserole that could serve as an entree for you and a side dish for the other guests. Do what feels right to you. Some hosts would be relieved and delighted to have your help; in other cases it wouldn't be appropriate. You will have to be the judge.

If you feel it simply isn't appropriate to inform your host of your food preferences or to bring your own dish, then you still have a couple of options:

Make do with what is available. Make a meal of the side dishes. A salad, some good bread, and a vegetable or two can be a wonderful meal. In fact, oftentimes, you'll find that it's all that you need to feel satisfied.

I sometimes choose this option even when I've told the host of my food preferences. If I feel as though it might be an imposition to have the host try to accommodate my needs, I may let the host know that no special effort has to be made on my behalf. I'll be fine with the side dishes. "Pam, I just wanted to let you know so that you won't have to fix a steak for me. But please don't worry; I'll have plenty to eat with everything else that you are making." "Are you sure?" "Oh, my, yes. I'll have more than enough with the salad, rolls, potato, and broccoli. Thanks so much."

That way, your host may know to make a little extra of a side dish or two, and he or she also has a warning and knows that you won't be eating the entree. From the perspective of the host, it might be disappointing to go to the trouble of preparing a dish only to find that you won't eat it.

Have a snack before you leave home. That way, you won't be as hungry, and it won't matter if you don't eat quite as much of your host's meal.

You Are the Host. What about when the tables are turned? You are the host, and you are accustomed to eating plant-based meals. Your guests, on the other hand, have traditional tastes and a traditional American eating style. Naturally, you want your guests to enjoy their meal. What should you prepare?

Again, you have options:

Your best bet is to make familiar favorites that just happen to be plant-based dishes and can be prepared according to your standards.

Some examples: your favorite pasta topped with a fresh marinara or tomato-based sauce, or tossed with a small amount of olive oil and some herbs—maybe some chopped fresh basil and Roma tomatoes. An alternative might be a colorful vegetable lasagna, or how about a meatless chili prepared with several different types of beans? All of these dishes could be served with a salad, good bread, and a light dessert, such as fruit sorbet or a dish of fresh berries dusted with powdered sugar.

These are foods that, while plant-based, are familiar enough to most people that they stand a good chance of being well-liked.

Another likely candidate is pizza, which can be topped with various sliced or chopped vegetables and a sprinkling of cheese (or it can be made without cheese). Burritos, tacos, and enchiladas can also be made with bean fillings, or even a combination of beans and another vegetable, such as chopped spinach or broccoli. If you use cheese, you can buy a low-fat cheese and use it lightly (since even low-fat cheese is relatively high in fat), or you may opt to leave the cheese out altogether.* If you are making bean burritos, try using black beans instead of pinto beans for a change of pace.

What? You don't cook? Then you might consider ordering food from a restaurant or caterer. If all else fails, you might consider going out to eat at a restaurant where everyone can order what they please.

---

*Fat-free cheese is an option for those who like it, but many people have strong negative opinions about the fat-free cheeses on the market. The primary complaints—it doesn't melt, and it has no flavor. My advice: don't force yourself to eat anything that you don't like.

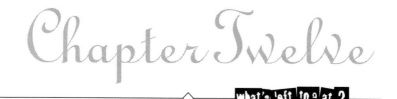

Chapter Twelve

Traveling Light

If you have the good fortune to travel for pleasure, or if you have to travel for work, then you are probably aware of the special challenges faced by travelers who want to eat well while they are away from home. Who hasn't had to find lunch at a truck stop along a highway or order a meal from an unfamiliar menu in a strange city?

Everybody is traveling today. Not only business people. Retirees who finally have the time to see the world, daytrippers toting backpacks and walking sticks, vacationers traveling by car with families, and adventure travelers spending a week in Timbuktu. I, too, am a frequent traveler, both for pleasure and for work, and I know that finding a way to eat well consistently while you are away from the controlled environment of your own home can be tough.

But it's possible…

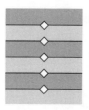

Your plane landed on time in Chicago;
    Have some Häagen-Dazs.
Your luggage landed ahead of schedule in Bolivia.
    Have some more.
        —From a magazine advertisement for Häagen-Dazs ice cream

Getting There
If By Land...

Remember the days of the family vacation? It was summertime—Mom and Dad in the front seat, bickering children in back, heading across country in the family Buick, no air conditioning and no sign of a rest stop for miles. I remember it well.

Times have changed, but some things stay the same. What can you pack in the cooler to take along in the car, or what do you eat along the way when your only choices are fast food and Stuckey's? Here are some suggestions if you are traveling by car (or bus), whether solo or en famille.

Cooler and Brown Bag Take-Alongs
Try these ideas, for starters:

- Fresh fruit (depending on the season, you might even pick some up along the way if you pass a roadside stand or farmers' market)
- Fruit salad—in cans with pop-up lids or made from fresh fruit and stored in an airtight, reusable container before you leave home
- Fresh vegetable pieces—bring along a bag of peeled baby carrots and a jar of salsa to use as dip. Bags of other pre-washed and cut fresh vegetables will also work, such as broccoli and cauliflower mixtures
- Homemade whole-grain muffins
- Bagels
- Ready-made deli containers of hummus (chickpea dip) for pita-pocket sandwiches and for a fresh vegetable dip
- Instant soup cups—add hot water, stir, and they're ready in five minutes. Get the hot water when you stop at a gas station.
- Instant hot cereal cups—just like the soup cups. At the time of writing, Fantastic Foods makes a wonderful line that is sold at supermarkets and natural foods stores.
- Homemade quick breads—zucchini, banana, and so on
- Homemade oatmeal cookies (they can be lower in fat when you make them yourself—see Chapter 16 for tips on modifying recipes)
- Graham crackers
- Canned vegetarian baked beans
- Single-serving, aseptically packaged boxes of fruit juice, fruit and vegetable juice blends, or soymilk
- Cans of fruit juice—these can be frozen before you leave and used to help keep other items cold in a bag or cooler. Drink the juice when it thaws.

- Peanut butter sandwiches made on whole-grain bread with a thin layer of peanut butter and slices of banana or apple
- Low-fat popcorn or pretzels
- Dried fruit
- Fig bars
- Cups of nonfat or soy yogurt

When people pack a bag lunch or a "cooler meal," they have a tendency to fall into the trap of thinking that there has to be a "main course," just like when they plan meals at home. A sandwich is often the focal point of a bag lunch, but it doesn't have to be. Mixing and matching some odds and ends can give you endless options. You may even find that it's more convenient to "graze" if you are traveling by car or bus, rather than having full meals, and that's fine.

If By Sea...

Cruising is almost synonymous with "feasting." Some of the best eating adventures can be had on cruise ships, but guilt doesn't have to be part of the experience. In fact, many ships now cater to people who are looking for a "healthful" vacation and offer a spa-like environment with food that is low in fat, saturated fat, and cholesterol or is vegetarian.

If you are planning a cruise, your best bet is to check with your travel agent or the customer services representative of the cruise line you are considering to ask for food service details. If you are really concerned about your meal options, or if you want to plan ahead, you may want to write to the cruise line and request sample menus and other meal information.

However, it's fairly easy to get healthful menu options on cruise ships these days. Some ships offer special menus for vegetarians or for people who want "healthful" choices, and many have items on the regular menu that are "flagged" if they meet certain criteria for being lower in fat and cholesterol. On some ships, the food is made to order, so you have the opportunity to make special requests about the way in which a dish is prepared.

In other cases, meals are served buffet-style. Cruise ship buffets are usually colossal spreads, and most contain a wide array of fresh fruits and vegetables. If entrees seem to be fat-rich and fiber-poor, pick and choose from the fruits, vegetables, and other side dishes to piece together a fabulous meal. But remember this tip for navigating cruise ship buffet lines: to steer clear of impulse choices and not-so-good-for-you temptations, survey the entire array of choices on the line and make a mental note of what you'll have before you walk through with your plate.

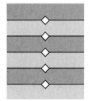 **"To eat healthfully, the passenger must become a prospector, digging out pure alternatives from a mountain of temptation."**
—Mark Seal in an article in the June 1996 issue of *Allure* magazine titled, "Airport 1996—The latest disaster isn't in the air—it's on the ground. Why is terminal food so...well, terminal?"

If By Air...

Air travel begins on land, at the airport—which, for me, remains one of the most exciting places around. I have memories of many a happy Saturday as a child dashing through Detroit's Metro Airport, reveling in the chaos inside the terminal while on my way to the observation deck where I spent hours watching the planes take off and land. It seemed as though all points on earth met there, with people from around the world converging momentarily in the same spot, only to be miles apart again a short time later, scattering in all directions for points around the globe. I daydreamed about stowing away and heading for someplace exotic. It was exhilarating.

The airport hasn't lost its sense of wonder for me as an adult. But as a frequent flyer, I've gained an appreciation for some of its amenities as well. Thank goodness for newsstands, where I can pick up a daily paper and the toothbrush I forgot to pack. Before take-off and during layovers, this is also where I might grab a quick snack or meal at a cafeteria, restaurant, food stand, or airline lounge.

How wide a range of food choices you'll find depends on the airport. Some tiny municipal airports offer little more than a few food stands—vending machines, at worst—whereas busier airports may have large food courts, restaurants, and cafeterias. Here's what to look for wherever you may be:

GOOD FOODS, BAD FOODS

Newsstands All but the smallest airports have them, but this is primarily a gum and candy bar scene. Of course I don't recommend snacking on candy. But if you are desperate, and it's candy that you want, go for the hard candies—lemon drops, butterscotch disks, peppermints. They're fat-free and low in calories, even if you eat a handful. No need to feel guilty about a few hard candies if they will hold you until you board the plane and your meal is served. Jellybeans and gumdrops are also good choices, relatively speaking.

If hard candies won't do it for you, then the next best choices are chocolate-covered raisins or peppermint patties. The fat in the thin layers of chocolate is balanced by the nearly-fat-free raisins and peppermint filling. Easy does it, though. Get the small bag of raisins.

Packages of cookies, crackers, nuts, and snack mixes at newsstands are generally all high in fat, so they're packed with calories. You may find fig bars or a small bag of gingersnaps or vanilla wafer cookies. These are usually relatively low in fat and are the best choices.

Read the nutrition label and aim for three grams of fat per serving or less. Make sure that the serving size is reasonable, though. If the serving size is tiny and you end up eating five servings' worth, you've defeated the purpose. Remember that even fat-free calories count, so if weight control is your issue, stick to the small, low-fat, single-serving snacks.

Unless you are trying to satisfy a sweet tooth, or if you need a more substantial snack, move on to some of the choices discussed next.

Food Stands My eyes lit up when I spotted the soft pretzel stand at Philadelphia International Airport. Pretzels—with or without mustard—are a good choice, low in fat and high in complex carbohydrates. At the time of writing, the pretzels served at the Philadelphia airport contain only about two grams of fat apiece and have 300 calories each.

Specialty food stands such as these have sprung up in airports everywhere. Frozen-yogurt stands are common, and many sell fat-free flavors. Frozen yogurt is an acceptable choice as a quick snack, with a couple of

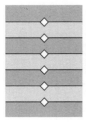

Helpful Hint...
Keep a small bag of dried fruit; whole-grain, low-fat crackers; or a little box of raisins with you when you travel. Grab an apple from the front desk as you check out of your hotel. You'll be sure to have something low-fat and nutritious on hand in case you need a fast snack later on when airport choices may be limited and more expensive.

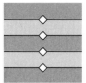

"The solution for healthy eating in airports is to bring your own fruit—apples, oranges, and bananas," says Justin Hayward of the forever-flying rock group the Moody Blues.

—From the article "Airport 1996" in *Allure* magazine, June 1996

caveats. First, choose a fat-free flavor instead of a flavor listed as "96% fat-free." The latter is made with whole milk, which is 4% fat by weight, hence the "96% fat-free." However, it's over 50% fat by calories—too much fat to be a good choice.

Second, take the yogurt but leave off the toppings. A decorative splash of sprinkles won't hurt—they're mostly sugar—and fruit topping is always a good choice. But steer clear of fattier toppings, such as hot fudge and chunks of peanut butter cup.

Candy and nut stands are ubiquitous. Follow the guidelines given earlier for newsstand candy choices. As for nuts and seeds, they are nearly all fat, so you won't want to eat them with abandon if you are concerned about your waistline. You may see dried fruit sold at candy and nut stands; it's a good choice and ounce-for-ounce lower in calories than nuts and seeds. Again, watch the portion size, since the calories can quickly add up. A handful will give you some quick energy without too many calories.

Combinations of nuts and dried fruits, or trail mix, can be fatty unless they consist primarily of fruit. Some also contain coconut, which is high in saturated fat and should be limited. The bottom line at candy and nut stands: go for the dried fruit or a handful of the fat-free candy choices noted earlier.

Gourmet coffee stands are another recent arrival at the airport. I am not an advocate of caffeine-containing beverages such as coffee, but one or two cups per day is not a problem for most people. If you lighten your coffee, use skim or low-fat milk or a nondairy creamer instead of whole milk or cream. A teaspoon or two in a cup of coffee will add a gram or two of fat, which isn't much.

Cappuccino, cafe latté, and cafe mocha are likely to contain a few grams of fat per cup if they are made with whole milk. Limit yourself to one cup.

Be extra careful about what you buy to go with your coffee. Commercially made muffins tend to be very high in fat. Take a peek at the paper lining the muffin tray. Do you see greasy spots? If so, it's a clue that those muffins are loaded with fat. The pastries are guaranteed to be high in fat, and much of that is saturated fat. Your best bet here is to take a biscotti, a dry, flavorful cookie that can be dunked in your coffee. Those that are not dipped in chocolate or that do not contain nuts are the lowest in fat. Otherwise, walk down to the cafeteria and buy a bagel.

You may see stands selling popcorn. Popcorn would be a great choice if you could be sure that it was popped in minimal oil or air popped. However, unless nutrition information is available at the stand (which I've never seen) and there are three grams of fat or less per three-cup serving, I recommend avoiding the popcorn, which probably has been made with copious amounts of fat.

Cafeterias Just like eating at a buffet on a cruise ship, when you eat in an airport cafeteria, it's a good practice to take a stroll down the line first to assess your choices. Airport cafeterias usually carry a smaller variety of cooked foods and more cold foods, packaged sandwiches, and grill items than do other cafeterias.

Generally, you'll find hot foods to be high in fat—hot dogs and French fries, for example. The pizza is loaded with fat, too, mostly due to greasy cheese and meat toppings. In circumstances where you would ordinarily get your food to order, you could ask that fatty toppings and part or all of the cheese be left off the pizza. At the airport, however, the pizza is ready-made; what you see is what you get.

You'll have more luck with the cold foods. This is a good opportunity to enjoy a fresh fruit salad, one of the best choices you can make. Another great choice is a mixed green salad; eat it with a fat-free dressing or squeeze a few lemon wedges on top and sprinkle on some black pepper. Have a roll or bagel with jelly if you are hungry for a little more.

People tend to skimp on fresh foods when they travel—especially fiber-rich fruits and vegetables—and to fill up on fast, processed foods instead, which are likely to be low in fiber and high in fat. Make it a habit to seek out fresh foods often. Many cafeterias place a bowl of fresh fruit near the check-out. Make it a habit to take a piece. Even if you don't eat it then, you can carry it and eat it later for a snack.

Other smart choices? Bottled fruit juices and waters are good. As with fresh fruits and vegetables, people tend to be neglect fluids when they travel. You'll feel better if you keep yourself well-hydrated.

Nonfat yogurt, plain or flavored, is fine; try eating it with some dry cereal if it's available or mix it into your fruit salad. Sandwiches tend to contain fatty fillings. You are better off picking up a few odds and ends to put together for a meal or snack. Keep in mind that a meal or snack doesn't have to have a "focal point" or main course. A meal made up of a bagel, a bottle of fruit juice, a bowl of fruit salad, and a small cup of yogurt, for instance, would be a smart choice.

Muffins and donuts are likely to be high in fat, so pass them up. Loaf bread, which may be able to be toasted, and bagels are great choices, low in fat and rich in complex carbohydrates. Eat them with jelly, which is fat-free, instead of margarine, butter, or cream cheese. If you prefer to put something on your bagel besides jelly, try mashed or sliced banana. Cinnamon-raisin bagels are my favorite, because they taste great with nothing on them.

Restaurants Some airports feature food courts to rival those at the largest shopping malls, with a range of restaurants including all of the major fast food chains and some conventional restaurants. We'll take a look at restaurant choices a little further on (also, see Chapter 10). The restaurants found in airports are essentially the same as those outside the airport.

Airline Lounges or Clubs Some frequent flyers have memberships in airline clubs that give them access to a quiet refuge during layovers. Here they have access to telephones and fax machines, newspapers, and refreshments.

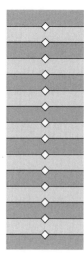

United Airlines scored tops in a survey of airline food offerings. United offers a vegetarian steak and pasta with just 3% of calories from fat, a vegetarian ravioli with only 9% of calories from fat, and a mixed-grain dish with 16% of calories from fat. None of the dishes contained cholesterol. An informal poll of nutrition experts also gave United top honors.

In a survey of 19 major airports across the U.S. and Canada, the best airports for availability of healthful foods were Los Angeles, Seattle, Pittsburgh, and Vancouver. The worst were Memphis, Dallas, Atlanta, and Phoenix, where travelers seeking low-fat or vegetarian food will find virtually nothing.

—From an October 1995 press release from the
Physicians Committee for Responsible Medicine

Airline clubs usually provide a range of hot and cold beverages, including soft drinks, tea, coffee, water, and juice. Some alcoholic drinks may also be available. Depending on the time of day, bagels and breakfast pastries may be set out, or there may be finger sandwiches and fresh fruit. Typically, you'll find cookies, crackers, snack mixes—sometimes chocolate candies.

Best choices? Settle back in a comfortable chair with a newspaper and a glass of mineral water with a wedge of lemon or lime. Fruit juices and flavored seltzer waters are other great choices. Herbal tea is another. Munch on some fresh vegetable crudités or fresh fruit, or have a bagel.

When choices are limited, remember that you probably won't have long to wait before you'll have another opportunity for a snack or meal—maybe on your upcoming flight. Only once in memory did my schedule end up such that I wasn't served a meal or snack all day long. Assess your choices at the time, and pick out the best ones. Ignore the rest.

A word about alcohol: I generally do not advocate alcoholic beverages, although, like coffee, a drink or two per day for those who enjoy it is usually not a problem. Alcohol is dehydrating, however, so if you indulge, make an extra effort to have water throughout the day as well.

In-Flight Meals My first peek behind the scenes of the airline industry came years ago when I visited the worksite of a friend who had relocated to Raleigh, N.C. to work with Sky Chefs, the food service company that catered the in-flight meals for American Airlines. I saw firsthand how meals were prepared on the tray lines, assembly-line fashion. Once ready, the trays of food were loaded onto carts designated for specific flights.

Like a scene from a science fiction movie, long lines of carts were suspended like a train from a track on the ceiling that snaked through the facility and carried the meals to the waiting planes. Later, in flight, the same carts would be rolled down the aisles of the planes during meal service and the trays served to passengers.

The actual assembly of the meals was also interesting. I remember seeing a tray line assembling the first-class meals for a Paris-bound flight and noting how elegant the trays looked. The dessert that night was cheesecake, served on lace doilies and china plates. I noticed the differences between foods served in the coach and first-class cabins. I also gained a better understanding of how special meal requests are handled.

My friend showed me the cycle menus that were being followed as well as additional menus for a surprisingly long list of special meals that were available. The place was buzzing with activity. The number of meals prepared each day was mind-boggling and the process required speed and coordination. Considering the complexity of the operation, I was impressed with the attention and care that went into handling the special meals. I gained a real appreciation of airline food service, and I've never looked at my in-flight meals in quite the same way again.

About Special Meals I've been ordering vegetarian meals on my flights for years. My meals always seem to look better than everyone else's. My friend at Sky Chefs explained to me that special meals usually get a little extra attention when they are prepared. I think the real answer is that my meal is more colorful than the others—full of brightly colored fruits and vegetables.

Some people aren't aware of the many options they have for special in-flight meals. Although each airline has its own list of choices, most offer diabetic, low-fat, low-cholesterol, low-sodium, Kosher, and vegetarian menus. Fruit plates are often available as well. Some overseas flights serve special ethnic meals for passengers of different cultures who frequent those flights. For instance, flights from the U.S. to London often offer Indian or Asian-style meals.

Vegetarian airline meals can usually be ordered two ways. A regular vegetarian meal contains no meat, fish or poultry, but it may contain dairy products and/or eggs. Vegetarian meals can also be ordered "vegan." A vegan meal contains no meat, fish or poultry, but it is also free of dairy products and eggs. Since vegan meals contain no animal products, they are cholesterol-free. They are usually lower in fat, too, since they are free of the eggs, milk, cheese, and other dairy products that can contribute a substantial amount of fat to the regular vegetarian meals.

Airline meals that are designated "low-fat, low cholesterol" are usually designed to contain 30% of calories from fat—too much fat for most of us. They are likely to be centered around a serving of meat, in keeping with the traditional American diet, so they are low in fiber.

You are better off with a vegan meal. Vegan meals are almost always very low in fat and high in fiber. Fat may be included on the tray in the form of salad dressing or a pat of margarine, but you can easily push that aside. Another excellent option is the fruit plate.

Ordering Special Meals At the time that you make your plane reservations, ask the agent if meals or snacks are scheduled to be served on any segments of your trip. If so, tell the agent that you want to request a special meal. Generally, special meal requests must be made within 24 hours of your flight. So if you forget to request a special meal when you make your reservation, you can call back later to place the order. Be sure to reconfirm your special meal order if you have to make a schedule change, since the agent might not automatically carry over the request.

Although the best meal choices are vegan (no dairy or eggs) or a fruit plate, you may have additional choices within the category of "vegetarian" if your destination takes you overseas. Now is your chance to experiment with some interesting ethnic cuisines. On a flight from the U.S. to Australia, I ordered "Hindu, no dairy" meals for a change of pace.

During Meal Service When meal service begins, you may need to tell your flight attendant that you ordered a special meal. Sometimes they will have identified you ahead of time; they might even check with you to confirm that you are expecting a special meal. Other times, you may be handed a regular meal unless you speak up and tell them that you are expecting something else.

What if they don't have my meal? There may be times that you won't receive the meal that you ordered. This can happen for a variety of reasons. If you have a last-minute change of schedule, there won't be enough time for an order to be processed, or if you have a change of aircraft for some reason, your meal won't follow you. If you are a business traveler upgrading from coach to first class at the last minute, the meal you ordered in coach may not be available for you in first class. Of course, sometimes you'll never know why your meal didn't make it. It can be frustrating at times, but mistakes happen, and you'll have to make the best of it.

If your meal doesn't show up, you have a number of options. You may want to take a regular meal and eat part of it. A lunch or dinner meal, for instance, will usually include a salad. If regular salad dressing is served with it, ask for a lemon wedge instead—you can improvise your own gourmet lemon juice and black pepper dressing. A roll or slice of bread is fine; leave off the butter. You might eat the rice and vegetables and leave the meat.

You might also ask the flight attendant to put something together for you based on what is on hand. On one flight, my flight attendant brought

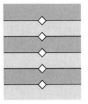

Helpful Hint...
If your flight attendant doesn't leave the entire can of juice or water with you, ask if you can have it. Don't be shy about asking for a second beverage, too, especially water. Ask for a piece of lemon or lime to flavor a glass of water or tomato juice.

me several wonderful whole grain flatbreads and a large plate of fresh fruits. If you are very hungry, you might ask for an extra regular meal so that you can have double servings of the bread, salad, vegetables, and so on. If a few more calories is what you are after, you can also ask for an extra beverage.

What About the Peanuts? Have you ever felt, "If I see one more peanut, I'm going to jump off this plane?" As I've noted before, peanuts are nearly all fat. Unless you are starving, just set them aside and enjoy your beverage.

And Beverage Service? Enjoy the beverage service—you need plenty of fluids when you fly. The best choices are nonalcoholic, non-caffeine-containing beverages such as mineral water, fruit juice, and tomato juice. Lemonade is fine, too.

Are You Really Hungry? One of my favorite airline souvenirs is an eyepatch that came in an overnight kit that I received on an overseas flight. With the kit came a sticker that could be affixed to your seat (at first, I thought it went on the eyepatch). The sticker reads: "Wake me for meals." I laugh every time I think of it.

As I noted earlier, only once in memory have I ever gone hungry while traveling by plane. It was a string of short flights with very little time between connections and no meals served in-flight. By the time I reached my destination that night, room service hours were over at my hotel, and all of the restaurants in town were closed. I ate a big breakfast the next day.

What's more likely to happen is that you'll be offered more food than you really need. You may have already eaten breakfast at home, for instance, and your morning flight serves another breakfast. On longer journeys, your eating schedule can get mixed up when you fly long distances and change time zones. You may be served meals at times when you aren't hungry.

Learn to pass on meals when you aren't hungry. Take a beverage instead, or just leave your tray table up and say, "no thanks." It's easy to overeat when you travel; when food is placed in front of you—and you're stuck there in your seat for another hour—it's not uncommon to find yourself munching on foods that you otherwise would not have eaten. Later, when you are hungry, you will probably be at your destination and can eat then. If not, you can reach for that piece of fresh fruit you've carried with you.

Once You're There: Restaurant Dining

We've already discussed strategies for eating out in restaurants in Chapter 10. You might also consider referring to *Vegetarian Journal's Guide to Natural Foods Restaurants in the* U.S. *and Canada* (Avery, 1993) if you are heading out to an unfamiliar city. The book is updated periodically and lists restaurants that are likely to offer plenty of healthful menu choices.

The following is also a quick reference to some good choices at several types of restaurants:

At Italian restaurants, try:

- Lentil or minestrone soup
- Pasta e fagioli (pasta and beans)
- Mixed green salads
- Fresh vegetable appetizers
- Pasta primavera
- Pasta with marinara sauce
- Plain Italian bread (dip it in a small amount of olive oil if weight control is not an issue for you)
- Cooked vegetables
- Fresh fruit for dessert (a fluted champagne glass filled with berries?)

At fast-food restaurants, try:

- Fruit juice
- Fat-free muffins
- Veggie burgers (skip the mayo and cheese)
- Bean burritos (ask for light cheese or skip it—you won't miss it)
- Bean soft tacos and bean tostadas (omit cheese as above)
- Pancakes with maple syrup (a relatively good breakfast choice, but skip the butter)

- English muffin with jelly
- Fresh vegetable sticks
- Low-fat salads
- Nonfat yogurt or skim milk
- Baked potato topped with salsa and chopped vegetables

At pizza shops, try:

- Cheeseless pizzas, or go light on the cheese
- Vegetable toppings: chopped green peppers and onions, mushrooms, tomato slices, yellow squash or zucchini, chopped broccoli and cauliflower, or pineapple chunks

At Mexican restaurants, try:

- Bean fillings (skip the cheese or ask the waiter to "go light" on it)
- Lettuce, tomato, onions, and salsa for toppings
- Gazpacho (a cold, spicy, tomato-based soup)
- Mixed green salad
- Steamed vegetables

At Indian restaurants, try:

- Dal (lentil soup) without added ghee (clarified butter)
- Vegetable curries
- Steamed rice
- Chappatti (bread) and papadum (ask for steamed, not deep-fried); menu listings for breads with the words "roti" or "nan" are usually baked or roasted, such as khasta roti or rogini nan.
- Chutneys
- Fresh exotic fruit
- Kachumbar (raw vegetables)

At Chinese restaurants, try:

- Vegetable soups or hot and sour soup
- Spring rolls instead of regular egg rolls
- Pot stickers (steamed vegetable dumplings)
- Chinese salads such as sweet and sour cabbage
- Sauteed greens (ask for minimal or no oil)
- Steamed rice
- Broccoli with garlic sauce, vegetable lo mein, Chinese mixed vegetables (ask for minimal or no oil)
- Fruit

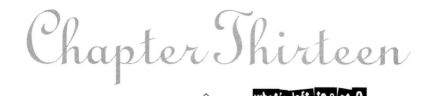

How to Get Support

It pays to have a plan in place if you are embarking on a journey. Likewise, when your goal is a lifestyle change, it's a good idea to have a plan, particularly one that includes plenty of support. Support can come in the form of people who can help you achieve your goals, a supportive living environment, books, videos, magazines, organizations, and other resources.

Get Educated

You need to educate yourself about nutrition and how to make effective dietary changes. This book is a good place to start, but there are other resources that will add dimension to what you've already learned. Sometimes it helps to hear the same information presented in different ways, by different people, or in different media. Repetition can assist you in learning and understanding, too.

To borrow Jeff Steingarten's phrase, the self-help/nutrition market—books, videos, and other products—is a "bloated juggernaut" that threat-

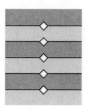

"Where are you going?" the cat asked.
"I don't know."
"Well, either road will get you there."
—The Cheshire Cat to Alice, who had lost her way.
From *Alice in Wonderland* by Lewis Carroll

ens to crush consumers, in many cases with information that is tainted by scientific inaccuracies and/or skewed by politics. Don't let yourself be stalled or sidetracked by materials that are, at best, a waste of time, or at worse, just plain nonsense. Let me assist you by sifting through the piles of nutrition-related educational materials and pointing out those that will be of most use.

The resource list that follows consists of sources of progressive, practical, accurate information to assist you in your efforts to change your eating style. While not exhaustive, it pinpoints some of the resources that, in my opinion, are the best.

Organizations

Center for Science in the Public Interest, Suite 300, 1875 Connecticut Avenue, N.W., Washington, D.C. 20009-5728; 202-332-9110. CSPI is an independent nonprofit consumer health group. Its *Nutrition Action Healthletter* accepts no government or industry funding.

National Center for Nutrition and Dietetics, The American Dietetic Association, 216 W. Jackson Blvd., Suite 800, Chicago, IL 60606-6995; 800-366-1655. This is the public education initiative of the ADA. Yes, the hotline is funded by industry dollars. But my suggestion is to call specifically for a free copy of the ADA's brochure, "Eating Well—the Vegetarian Way," as well copies of the ADA's position paper on vegetarian diets and its vegetarian nutrition fact sheet. These materials are sound. The ADA referral service can also give you the names and phone numbers of nutritionists in your area who profess to specialize in plant-based diets.

Physicians Committee for Responsible Medicine, 5100 Wisconsin Ave, N.W., Suite 400, Washington, D.C. 20016; 202-686-2210. While often attacked by mainstream medical organizations for objecting to the use of animals in scientific experimentation and its "vegetarian agenda," I find this organization's nutrition-related materials to be some of the most progressive. Ask for a copy of "The New Four Food Groups."

Vegetarian Nutrition Dietetic Practice Group, Division of Practice, The American Dietetic Association (address above). This is an interest group of the ADA for members who specialize in or want to learn more about plant-based diets. Among other activities, the group publishes the quarterly newsletter, *Issues in Vegetarian Dietetics*. The newsletter and other educational materials produced by the practice group are also available to non-members.

The Vegetarian Resource Group, P.O. Box 1463, Baltimore, MD 21203; 410-366-8343. The nonprofit VRG is the leading source of reliable, progressive materials about plant-based diets. All nutrition and health-related materials are peer-reviewed by registered dietitians and physicians who are knowledgeable about plant-based diets. The group publishes the bimonthly Vegetarian Journal.

Books About Plant-Based Diets

Becoming Vegetarian, by Vesanto Melina, R.D.; Brenda Davis, R.D.; and Victoria Harrison, R.D.; Book Publishing Company, Summertown, Tenn., 1995.

Being Vegetarian, by Suzanne Havala, M.S., R.D., for the American Dietetic Association. Chronimed Publishing, Minneapolis, Minn., 1996.

Dr. Dean Ornish's Program for Reversing Heart Disease, by Dean Ornish, M.D. Random House, New York, N.Y., 1990.

Eat More, Weigh Less, by Dean Ornish, M.D. HarperCollins Publishers, New York, N.Y., 1995.

Shopping for Health: A Nutritionist's Aisle-by-Aisle Guide to Smart, Low-fat Choices at the Supermarket, by Suzanne Havala, M.S., R.D. HarperPerennial, New York, N.Y., 1996.

Simple, Lowfat & Vegetarian, by Suzanne Havala, M.S., R.D.; and Mary Clifford, R.D. The Vegetarian Resource Group, Baltimore, Md., 1994.

The Vegetarian Way, by Virginia Messina, M.P.H., R.D., and Mark Messina, Ph.D. Crown Trade Paperbacks, New York, N.Y., 1996.

Vegan Handbook, Debra Wasserman and Reed Mangels, Ph.D., R.D. The Vegetarian Resource Group, Baltimore, Md., 1996.

Vegetarian Times Vegetarian Beginner's Guide, by the editors of Vegetarian Times magazine. MacMillan, New York, N.Y., 1996.

For children and teens

A *Teen's Guide to Going Vegetarian*, by Judy Krizmanic. Viking, New York, N.Y., 1994.

Dr. Attwood's Low-Fat Prescription for Kids, by Charles Attwood, M.D., with foreword by Benjamin Spock, M.D. Viking, N.Y., New York, 1995. (Note: while there is still insufficient scientific data upon which to base recommendations that Western children should consume a very low-fat diet, this book contains information that is generally helpful and progressive in an area—nutrition for children—for which there is very little reliable printed material available.)

Cookbooks

This section is a toughie, because there are so many good cookbooks on the market now that focus on plant-based dishes. I've whittled this list down to several good starter cookbooks. Note that I do not list some of my sentimental favorites because of their heavy use of dairy products and eggs, hence the higher saturated fat and cholesterol composition of their recipes.

All-purpose cookbooks:

Lean, Luscious and Meatless, by Bobbie Hinman and Millie Snyder. Prima Publishing, Rocklin, Calif., 1992.

The Meatless Gourmet: Easy Lowfat Favorites, by Bobbie Hinman. Prima Publishing, Rocklin, Calif., 1997.

The Meatless Gourmet, by Bobbie Hinman, Prima Publishing, Rocklin, Calif., 1995.

The New Laurel's Kitchen, by Laurel Robertson, Carol Flinders, and Brian Ruppenthal. Ten Speed Press, Berkeley, Calif., 1986.

New Vegetarian Cuisine, by Linda Rosensweig and the food editors of *Prevention* magazine. Rodale Press, Emmaus, Pa., 1994.

The Peaceful Palate, by Jennifer Raymond. Heart and Soul Publications, Calistoga, Calif., 1992.

Simply Vegan, by Debra Wasserman. The Vegetarian Resource Group, Baltimore, Md., 1994, Fifth Edition.

Table for Two, by Joanne Stepaniak. Book Publishing Company, Summertown, Tenn., 1996.

The Uncheese Cookbook, by Joanne Stepaniak. Book Publishing Company, Summertown, Tenn., 1996.

Vegan Vittles, by Joanne Stepaniak. Book Publishing Company, Summertown, Tenn., 1996.

Vegetarian Times Complete Cookbook, by the editors of Vegetarian Times magazine. MacMillan, New York, N.Y., 1995.

The Complete Soy Cookbook, by Paulette Mitchell. Macmillan, N.Y., 1998.

Fabulous Beans by Barb Bloomfield. Book Publishing Company, Summertown, Tenn., 1994.

The Savory Way: High Spirited, Down-to-Earth Recipes from the Author of The Greens Cookbook, by Deborah Madison, Bantam Books, New York, N.Y., 1990.

Soy of Cooking: Easy-to-Make Vegetarian, Low-Fat, Fat-Free & Antioxidant-Rich Recipes by Marie Oser. Chronimed Publishing, Minneapolis, Minn., 1996.

Vegetarian Cooking for Everyone by Deborah Madison, Broadway Books, New York, N.Y., 1997.

1,000 Vegetarian Recipes by Carol Gelles. Macmillan, New York, N.Y., 1996.

For children:

Leprechaun Cake and Other Tales, by Vonnie Crist and Debra Wasserman. The Vegetarian Resource Group, Baltimore, Md. 21203, 1995.

Magazines and Newsletters

Environmental Nutrition newsletter, P.O. Box 420451, Palm Coast, FL 32142-0451. 800-829-5384.

Nutrition Action Healthletter (see Center for Science in the Public Interest above).

Vegetarian Journal (see The Vegetarian Resource Group above).

Vegetarian Times magazine, P.O. Box 570, Oak Park, IL 60303; 708-848-8100 or 800-435-9610.

Web Sites

The American Dietetic Association http://www.eatright.org

Center for Science in the Public Interest (CSPI) http://www.cspinet.org

The Vegetarian Resource Group www.vrg.org

Other Materials

Mediterranean Food Pyramid, available from Oldways Preservation and Exchange Trust, 45 Milk Street, Boston, MA 02109; 617-695-2300. Other culture-specific food guides are also available, emphasizing the healthiest choices within those cultures' eating patterns (Asian, Latin American, and so on).

Shopping for Health video series by Suzanne Havala, M.S., R.D., and Leni Reed, M.P.H., R.D. Smart choices at the supermarket. Series includes Shopping for Health (core tape), Shopping for Women's Health, Shopping for Heart Health, Shopping for Health: Weight Management. For information write to Shopping for Health, P.O. Box 221383, Charlotte, N.C., 28222-1383.

The Vegetarian Food Pyramid, Health Connections, 55 West Oak Ridge Dr., Hagerstown, Md., 21740; 800-543-8700.

Get Involved

There are many ways to educate yourself about how to make dietary lifestyle changes. In addition to gathering reliable resources, you might consider immersing yourself in the following activities:

Community support groups. Appropriate groups might be hidden behind the guise of a cardiac rehabilitation program or cancer recovery program, probably affiliated with your local hospital, a medical clinic, or a nonprofit agency. Some community hospitals are developing "mind-body" programs that incorporate a nutrition/wellness component. If nothing is available in your area, you might consider organizing your own group, even if you begin with only three or four people.

Local vegetarian societies. Many local vegetarian groups hold monthly potluck get-togethers, and some sponsor restaurant outings. Attending these dinners is a great way to sample new dishes and to be inspired by the varieties, colors, flavors, and aromas of healthful, plant-based meals. To find a local vegetarian organization, inquire at your neighborhood natural foods store or check the Yellow Pages. You can also call the Vegetarian Resource Group (address and phone listed earlier) for a list of vegetarian organizations in your state or city.

Advocate for yourself and others. It will be easier for all of us to get healthful foods in our supermarkets, restaurants, and schools if we each do our part to lobby for the necessary changes.

Organizations such as the Center for Science in the Public Interest and the Vegetarian Resource Group often urge their members to act on issues concerning legislation or regulation change by assisting with letter-writing campaigns. You can also help on the local level by taking the time to tell supermarket managers about products you'd like to see stocked at the store. Tell chefs and restaurant owners about dishes you'd like to see on their menus, and insist that schools offer healthful alternatives in their cafeterias.

Join a food co-op. Food co-ops can be good sources of locally grown organic produce during the growing season. You'll save money on other products, too, especially higher-priced, natural food brands, since co-ops buy in volume.

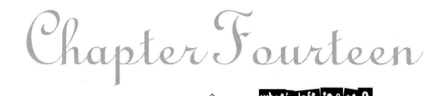

Chapter Fourteen

what's left to eat ?

A Simple Meal-Planning Guide

Refer to the Smart Daily Food Guide that follows to help you plan your meals or to assist you in evaluating your diet. Adults should aim for at least the minimum number of servings from each food group daily. If you are very athletic and need more calories, or if your calorie needs are increased for other reasons, such as pregnancy or breastfeeding, you should eat a greater number of servings from all of the groups to meet your calorie needs.

You'll note that I've made this food guide meat-free, or vegetarian, with optional, limited amounts of dairy products and egg whites. Dairy products were included, but not necessarily encouraged, simply because they are a concentrated source of calcium, a key nutrient of issue for many women in this country. As I've described earlier, the issue of recommendations for calcium is fraught with complexities, but some people who do tolerate dairy products may wish to use them as a dependable calcium source. If you do use dairy products, choose nonfat varieties. Over two-thirds of the fat in dairy products is saturated fat.

A limited number of optional egg whites has also been included for those who would like to use them in baking or as a binder in some recipes. Substitutes for eggs in baking, however, are discussed in Chapter 16. For those who are not yet ready to dispense with meats entirely, my suggestion is to buy the leanest forms you can find and use them only as a minor ingredient in a dish or as a condiment. If you do choose to eat meat, small servings of fish are the best choice.

If your diet consists of nothing but plant matter, you should take a supplement of vitamin B12—or eat vitamin B12-fortified foods—to be on the safe side. Also, if you do not consume dairy products and have limited exposure to sunlight, a vitamin D supplement of not more than 100% of the RDA may be indicated. A registered dietitian or your health care provider can help assess your individual needs.

A Smart Daily Food Guide
Food Group Daily Servings Serving Sizes

Breads and cereals—6 or more
- 1 slice bread
- 1/2 bun, English muffin, or bagel
- 1/2 pita pocket
- 1 flour tortilla
- 1 oz. dry cereal
- 1/2 cup cooked cereal
- 1/2 cup cooked rice or other grains
- 1/2 cup cooked pasta

Vegetables—4 or more
- 1/2 cup cooked or 1 cup raw
- 3/4 cup vegetable juice

Legumes and plant products—
- 2 to 3 1/2 cup cooked beans, high protein peas, or lentils
- 8 ounces soymilk
- 4 ounces tofu or tempeh
- 1 1/2 ounces soy cheese
- 2 Tablespoons nuts, seeds, or nut and seed butters
- 3-ounce veggie burger patty or 1 vegetarian hot dog

Fruits—3 or more
- 1 medium piece fresh fruit
- 1/2 cup fruit juice
- 1/2 cup canned or cooked fruit
- 2 Tablespoons dried fruit

GOOD FOODS, BAD FOODS

Optional

Dairy products—Limit 2
- 8 ounces nonfat yogurt or nonfat milk
- 1 ounce nonfat cheese

Egg whites—Limit 2–4
- 2–4 egg whites

Fats—Limit as much as possible; choose olive oil or canola oil if you add fat to your food, or buy spreads with the least amount of saturated fat

Sweets—Limit as much as possible; choose nonfat sweets when you want something sweet

Alcohol—If you don't drink, don't start. If you do drink, limit yourself to fewer than two drinks per day, but only if your physician or health care provider indicates that it is acceptable for you to use alcohol. Pregnant women, children, and adolescents should abstain.

Making Great Choices

If I've characterized the mainstream nutrition community's dietary message as "anything goes," then there's also an opposite extreme to that picture. That is, some people still envision a dietitian as a finger-wagging dietary policewoman (in a hairnet) who takes all of the fun out of eating. The message that some people hear when they speak to a professional about their diet or they read about nutrition in the news is, "Don't eat this, don't eat that." The "don'ts" seem to overshadow the "do's" and leave many people with absolutely no idea of what they can fix for dinner tonight.

I wrote *Shopping for Health* in 1996 for that reason—to give people lots of ideas of healthful, good-tasting foods that they can put into their grocery carts when they shop. The emphasis is on the positive in order to help make readers aware that, far from being limited, a healthful diet includes many, many satisfying food choices.

In a more general way, the information that follows should help you see just how many good choices there are within the various food groups that make up the foundation of the Smart Daily Food Guide:

Breads and Cereals

Eat a minimum of six servings a day. Choose whole-grain products as often as possible.

If all you can envision is whole-wheat bread and bran flakes, widen your view. Mixed grain breads are delicious and so much more flavorful than the soft white kind. Think oats, rye, millet, sprouted wheat, and amaranth. Make your own bread—use a bread machine if you lack time or elbow grease. When you make your own bread, you can create all sorts of wonderful combinations of whole grains, and you can toss in some chopped dried fruits, nuts, and spices for a change of pace.

Try whole-wheat pita pockets, whole-grain flat breads, and whole-grain muffins. If you make your own muffins at home—they're very easy and quick to make—you can cut back on the oil in the recipe. Bake a batch of muffins, and if you can't eat them all right away, freeze the rest to take out as you need.

Try hot whole-grain cooked cereal for breakfast. Multigrain hot cereals are delicious and, like breads, can be made in variations that incorporate chopped dried fruit, nuts, and cinnamon. Let hot cereal cook overnight in a crockpot while you sleep so that it will be ready when you are in the morning. Live alone? There are little versions of the classic big crockpot that are just right for one or two people. Hot cereal topped with applesauce or sliced fresh fruit is also good.

Also experiment with traditional grains of other cultures, such as millet, amaranth, spelt, and quinoa (pronounced keen' wah). Add a handful of barley or bulgur wheat to soups and stews.

Then there's rice. Have you tried jasmine rice? Basmati? Arborio? If you haven't, put them at the top of your grocery list. They come in "brown" rice varieties as well as the regular white varieties. Jasmine rice has a wonderful aroma, and basmati rice has a delicious, nutty flavor.

Pasta. There are whole-grain varieties in most supermarkets, but you may have to look in the "health food" section of the store to find them. If you've tried whole-grain pasta and don't care for it, there's no need to fret. Every grain product that you eat does not have to be a whole-grain product. In the case of pasta, you may prefer the traditional white-flour pasta, and that's fine.

A piece of advice, though: Buy pasta that is made without egg yolks. Egg noodles contain a hefty amount of cholesterol. Pastas made without egg yolk are very easy to find—they are the most prevalent type in super-markets. Have you tried couscous? It's a Middle Eastern pasta—tiny round pieces of semolina—that is quick-cooking. You can serve it topped with cooked vegetables as a main dish or even tossed with bits of dried fruit as a side dish.

Vegetables

Eat at least four servings a day. That's easier than it sounds. If you consider that half a cup is a serving of a cooked vegetable, a good-sized portion at a meal could easily equal one cup. If your diet is plant-based, and grains, fruits, vegetables, and legumes are the foundation of your diet, then you'll find that four servings a day can easily be met, often in one meal.

Concerning vegetables, it doesn't matter if they're fresh, frozen, or canned. If you buy canned vegetables, you can rinse them in a colander to remove most of the salt. Fresh and frozen vegetables are the most nutri-tious, since the heat of canning can destroy some vitamins, and some vit-amins and minerals are leached out into the water packed with the veg-etables in the can. Nevertheless, it's fine to include some canned vegetables in your diet for convenience and a change of pace. Just because they aren't as nutritious as fresh or frozen doesn't mean that they have no value.

When you shop for fresh vegetables in the supermarket, do you make a beeline for the iceberg lettuce, tomatoes, and bananas and bypass every-thing else? If so, you are missing some terrific choices.

Make a pact with yourself to spend a little extra time looking at every-thing there is and experimenting with some items you've never before tried. Most produce managers are more than happy to explain how to choose and prepare the items they stock if you are feeling less than confident. Some good places to start: Try fresh kale sauteed with a drop of olive oil and some minced garlic; have a baked sweet potato topped with a bit of brown sugar or crushed pineapple and drizzled with fresh lime juice; steam some broccoflower; cut some jicama into matchstick-sized pieces for sal-ads or just to munch on.

If all you can envision when you step into the produce section is wash-ing, peeling, and chopping—lots of work—you may be a candidate for some "convenience" vegetables. You may pay more if someone else peels your carrots for you or washes and mixes your salad greens, but it may be worth it. Try peeled baby carrots dipped into salsa or hummus (garbanzo bean dip) for a nutritious and tasty snack. Buy prewashed baby spinach leaves for salads, and if they begin to spoil before you can use them in salad, steam them in the microwave or in a skillet and eat them as wilted spinach instead. Buy ready-to-eat, fresh vegetable mixtures such as broccoli, cauliflower, carrots, and peapods to make a quick stir-fry over rice.

For some of the best-tasting and most nutrient-packed vegetables, stop at a farmers' market or roadside stand during the growing season. Buying seasonal produce grown locally and, often, organically, is the best choice of all.

Legumes and High-Protein Plant Products

Choose two or three servings of these foods each day. It's easy to do, since only a half cup counts as a serving. When I fix a mixed green salad for myself, I usually add one cup of garbanzo beans to it, among other things. Voila! That's two servings of legumes right there. Vegetarian chili? One cup is a typical serving. That counts as two servings of legumes.

Legumes, or dried beans and peas, come in many shapes, colors, and sizes. Think kidney beans, black-eyed peas, black beans, pinto beans, cannelloni beans, navy beans, and split peas. Think chili, Hoppin' John, black beans and rice, black bean burritos, pasta e fagioli, navy bean soup, split pea soup, bean dip, bean salad, and baked beans, to name only a few.

Don't forget the lentils. When my Indian friend first took me to the Indian market where she shops, I was astounded to learn that there were so many different types of lentils. Red, black, orange, brown, yellow. They were beautiful. We don't see most of these varieties in the regular American supermarket. My friend explained to me that often before leaving for work in the morning, she turns her crockpot on to low heat and puts in a few cups of water and a couple of handfuls of different types of lentils. To that she adds whatever leftover vegetables she has from dinner the night before. This cooks all day, and when she comes home from work, she has lentil stew over steamed rice with a piece of Indian bread.

Dried beans, peas, and lentils are some of the most versatile foods around. However, if you buy them in their dry form, you have to soak them for several hours (or overnight) until they are soft enough to cook, or you have to prepare them in a pressure cooker. (An exception is lentils and split peas, which are often small enough that they can simmer for a couple of hours and be soft enough to eat.) I live in the South, where many people still soak their beans, while my Indian friend is in the habit of cooking dried beans in one of her small, skillet-sized Indian pressure cookers.

I, on the other hand, buy canned beans, which are ready to use. Nutritionally, canned beans are perfectly acceptable; you can rinse them in a colander to remove the salt. Nothing beats the convenience. I've been known to heat up some black beans out of a can, top them with a little salsa and, with a couple of slices of whole wheat toast, call it dinner. A gourmet meal it's not, but it is a healthful and delicious one.

Soy foods are another great option. Did you know that you can buy canned soybeans now in many natural-foods stores and some supermarkets? Most people, however, are more familiar with soybeans in their processed forms, such as tofu. Tofu can be cut up into cubes and used in stir-fries, but I prefer using tofu in some less traditional ways.

Try tofu in place of eggs to make a tofu-salad sandwich, or make "scrambled tofu" for breakfast or as a sandwich filling in a pita pocket or a bakery roll. Use tofu to make pudding, quiche, pie fillings—even tofu cheesecake—all with much less total fat and saturated fat than their egg-and-dairy-laden counterparts, and no cholesterol. Experiment with recipes from some of the soy cookbooks available in bookstores. Louise Hagler's *Tofu Cookery* is a classic—the photographs are astounding (but cut back on the oil in the recipes)—or give Marie Oser's *Soy of Cooking* a try.

There are many other soy products that are well worth trying. Soymilk is a delicious alternative to cow's milk and is a great idea for anyone who is lactose intolerant. It is available fortified with calcium, vitamin D, and vitamin B12. It has a slight beany aftertaste that I personally find appealing. I usually buy the vanilla-flavored variety, and I use it on my cereal every morning. Soymilk can be used cup for cup in place of cow's milk in any recipe. Soy cheese and soy yogurt are also available in natural foods stores.

Many people find that vegetarian burger patties, veggie hot dogs, and other soy- or vegetable-based meat analogs are convenient and great-tasting. This type of product was once found only in natural foods stores, but for the past few years, retailers have been vying for space in the regular supermarket as the popularity of these products has skyrocketed.

You might think you would find products like these in the meat case next to their real-meat counterparts. Instead, you'll usually find them in the frozen-food case near the breakfast items—waffles and egg substitutes. These products come in many, many varieties. Some have several grams of fiber, and all are lower in fat and saturated fat than their meat counterparts and are cholesterol-free. Kids love them, and they make a quick and easy food item to have on hand for teens for meals or snacks.

Nuts, seeds, and nut and seed butters can also be grouped with the legumes and high-protein plant products, but they differ from most of the other foods in this group in that most of their calories come from fat. Adults who want to control their weight should go easy on nuts and seeds, since fat is such a concentrated source of calories. A sprinkling here and there in a salad or stir-fry is fine.

Children and other people with high-calorie needs can use nuts and seeds more freely—peanut butter on crackers or on an apple as a snack, for example, or dried fruit and nuts in a trail mix.

Fruits

Choose three or more servings daily. One medium-sized piece of fruit is a serving, as is half a cup of fruit juice or canned fruit. Canned fruit is lower in fiber than fresh fruit, since the peel has been removed, and fruit juice is nearly devoid of fiber. So be sure to choose fresh fruit often in order to get plenty of fiber and other beneficial phytochemicals that may be more available in fresh fruit.

Just as you should experiment with a wide variety of vegetables, look carefully at the fruit the next time you shop, and try something that you've never tasted before. Mangoes and papayas are becoming commonplace in American supermarkets, and they are nutritional superstars. Think of it this way: What's the worst that could happen if you bought a new food and didn't like it? And the chances are very good that you'll find some new favorites.

Keep several types of fresh fruit on hand at home. Get into the habit of carrying a piece of fruit in the car when you are out for the day, in your brief-case, or in your bag lunch. At home, if fruit is getting close to spoiling before you can eat it, it's a good time to make a fruit salad.

Chopped fresh fruit is delicious in hot cereal. And here's one you've probably never tried: salad dressing made from nothing but fresh fruit. I know someone who blenderizes a seeded tangerine with a chunk of apple and pours the mixture over her salad. It's fresh and sweet and far more nutritious than bottled salad dressing.

Remember to stop at the farmers' market or roadside stands, too, for seasonal, locally grown fruit.

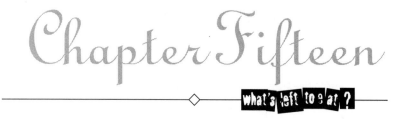

Chapter Fifteen

◇ ━━ what's left to eat ? ━━

Menus Made Easy

It takes practice and time to feel comfortable with new dietary habits. So if you find yourself stumped when it comes to putting a meal together, you aren't alone. Most people find that planning meals becomes easier as they master and refine their new skills.

For now, take heart and look over the menus that follow for ideas. All of these menus are created without the use of animal products. If you choose to substitute or add eggs, dairy products, or meat, refer to the guidelines in the last chapter.

Menu items listed are suggestions only. You'll find recipes for these and other healthful, plant-based dishes in the cookbooks listed in Chapter 13.

Draw up a list of some of your favorite foods and work them into menus of your own. The next chapter, which includes information about modifying your favorite recipes, may also stimulate your creativity. Enjoy!

Begin with breakfast. The menus that follow comprise traditional American breakfast foods, but don't let that stop you from being a little more creative if you are so inclined. Miso soup and rice is a fine way to start the day, and a bowl of cereal can also be a perfectly acceptable snack or supper, too.

Menu One
- 1 cup cooked oatmeal with cinnamon, raisins, and 2 Tbsp. wheat germ
- 8 oz. fortified soymilk, vanilla flavored
- 2 slices whole-wheat toast brushed with olive oil and with
- 2 Tbsp. fruit preserves
- 1/2 grapefruit

  Calories: 604 – Fat (grams): 12 – Percent calories from fat: 18

  Saturated fat (grams): 1 – Cholesterol (mg): 0 – Dietary fiber (grams): 10

  Protein (grams): 18 – Sodium (mg): 413 – Iron (mg): 4 – Calcium (mg): 242

Menu Two
- 6 oz. calcium-fortified orange juice
- 2 slices eggless French toast with
- 1/2 cup blueberry compote and maple syrup
- Sliced banana

  Calories: 686 – Fat (grams): 10 – Percent calories from fat: 13

  Saturated fat (grams): 1 – Cholesterol (mg): 0 – Dietary fiber (grams): 9

  Protein (grams): 12 – Sodium (mg): 441 – Iron (mg): 5 – Calcium (mg): 175

Menu Three
- 6 oz. prune juice
- 1/2 cup apricot-applesauce
- 2 raisin bran muffins
- 6 oz. flavored soy yogurt

  Calories: 608 – Fat (grams): 15 (less, if muffins are homemade using less oil)

  Percent calories from fat: 22 – Saturated fat (grams): 2 – Cholesterol (mg): 42 (none, if muffins are homemade using egg substitute) – Dietary fiber (grams): 9 – Protein (grams): 16 – Sodium (mg): 399 – Iron (mg): 5 – Calcium (mg): 177

Menu Four

- 1 1/2 cup whole-grain flake cereal with
- 8 oz. fortified soymilk, vanilla flavored
- 2 slices whole-wheat toast brushed with olive oil and with
- 2 Tbsp. fruit-only preserves
- 1/2 cup fresh fruit salad

   Calories: 581 – Fat (grams): 11 – Percent calories from fat: 17

   Saturated fat (grams): 1 – Cholesterol (mg): 0 – Protein (grams): 19

   Dietary fiber (grams): 15 – Sodium (mg): 970 – Iron (mg): 19 – Calcium (mg): 239

Menu Five

- 1 cup hot multigrain cereal with 1/4 cup chopped dried fruit and 2 tsp. brown sugar
- 8 oz. fortified soymilk, vanilla flavored
- 1 oatmeal muffin
- 6 oz. calcium-fortified orange juice

   Calories: 657 – Fat (grams): 9 – Percent calories from fat: 12

   Saturated fat (grams): 1 – Cholesterol (mg): 21 (none, if muffins are made with egg

   substitute) – Protein (grams): 16 – Dietary fiber (grams): 5 – Sodium (mg): 801

   Iron (mg): 5 – Calcium (mg): 274

Menu Six

- 1/2 cup stewed prunes
- Sliced banana
- 2 whole-grain waffles with maple syrup
- 6 oz. grapefruit juice

   Calories: 655 – Fat (grams): 8 – Percent calories from fat: 11

   Saturated fat (grams): 0 – Cholesterol (mg): 0 – Protein (grams): 8

   Dietary fiber (grams): 7 – Sodium (mg): 587 – Iron (mg): 7 – Calcium (mg): 125

Menu Seven

- 1/2 cup scrambled tofu with 1/2 cup sauteed green peppers and onions, topped with 2 Tbsp. salsa
- 2 slices multigrain toast brushed with 1 Tbsp. fruit preserves
- 3/4 cup fat-free hash-brown potatoes
- 6 oz. orange-pineapple juice

   Calories: 660 – Fat (grams): 14 – Percent calories from fat: 19
   Saturated fat (grams): 2.5 – Cholesterol (mg): 0 – Protein (grams): 30
   Dietary fiber (grams): 10 – Sodium (mg): 466 – Iron (mg): 17 – Calcium (mg): 334

Easy Ideas for Light Meals

Note that in the nutritional analyses that follow these menus (as well as main meal menus), the sodium levels are often quite high due to the use of salty commercial soups and canned beans in the computer database used to analyze the menus. Sodium levels can be drastically reduced when canned beans are rinsed before using and when "no salt added" canned soups and canned tomato products are used in meal preparation.

Menu One

- Large mixed-green salad topped with 3/4 cup garbanzo beans, sliced Roma tomato, 3 black olives, splash of balsamic vinegar, and freshly grated black pepper
- Baked potato topped with 3/4 cup thick lentil soup
- Water with lemon

   Calories: 343 – Fat (grams): 6 – Percent calories from fat: 16
   Saturated fat (grams): 1 – Cholesterol (mg): 5 – Protein (grams): 16 – Dietary fiber (grams): 10 – Sodium (mg): 1,241 (much less if soup is homemade without salt and if beans are rinsed before adding to salad) – Iron (mg): 6 – Calcium (mg): 130

Menu Two

- 1 cup vegetarian chili over
- 1 cup steamed brown rice
- 3/4 cup cooked kale with minced garlic and sesame seeds
- 3/4 cup steamed corn
- Fresh pear slices
- Water with lime

   Calories: 706 – Fat (grams): 5 – Percent calories from fat: 6 – Saturated fat (grams): 0
   Cholesterol (mg): 0 – Protein (grams): 27 – Dietary fiber (grams): 26 – Sodium (mg):
   960 (less if chili is homemade and beans are rinsed) – Iron (mg): 8 – Calcium (mg): 232

Menu Three

- Vegetarian burger patty on an English muffin with lettuce, tomato, alfalfa sprouts, and soy mayo/mustard sauce
- 3/4 cup marinated bean salad
- Cranberry juice with seltzer water

   Calories: 391 – Fat (grams): 4 – Percent calories from fat: 9
   Saturated fat (grams): 0 – Cholesterol (mg): 0 – Protein (grams): 23
   Dietary fiber (grams): 10 – Sodium (mg): 977 – Iron (mg): 6 – Calcium (mg): 204

Menu Four

- 1 cup tomato-rice soup
- Mock egg salad sandwich (tofu salad made with reduced-fat tofu; on toasted rye bread)
- Green pepper, celery, and carrot sticks with hummus dip
- Orange wedges
- Water with lemon

   Calories: 453 – Fat (grams): 11 – Percent calories from fat: 22
   Saturated fat (grams): 1 – Cholesterol (mg): 0 – Protein (grams): 14
   Dietary fiber (grams): 12 – Sodium (mg): 1,376 (much less if soup is homemade without salt) – Calcium (mg): 191

Menu Five

- Black-bean burrito with salsa
- 3/4 cup tomato-cucumber salad
- Papaya slices with freshly squeezed lime juice
- Flavored seltzer water

   Calories: 333 – Fat (grams): 4 – Percent calories from fat: 11

   Saturated fat (grams): 0 – Cholesterol (mg): 0 – Protein (grams): 14

   Dietary fiber (grams): 8 – Sodium (mg): 132 – Iron (mg): 5 – Calcium (mg): 144

Menu Six

- 1 cup navy-bean soup
- Tomato sandwich on toasted dark rye bread with pesto spread
- 3/4 cup vinaigrette cole slaw
- Fresh apple
- Water with lemon

   Calories: 427 – Fat (grams): 9 – Percent calories from fat: 19

   Saturated fat (grams): 2 – Cholesterol (mg): 0 – Protein (grams): 15

   Dietary fiber (grams): 12 – Sodium (mg): 1,326 (much less if soup is homemade

   without salt) – Calcium (mg): 188

Menu Seven

- 1 cup black-bean soup with chopped onions
- Whole-grain pita pocket filled with garbanzo bean spread, shredded carrot, and alfalfa sprouts
- 1/2 cup fruit sorbet
- Water with lime

   Calories: 443 – Fat (grams): 6 – Percent calories from fat: 12

   Saturated fat (grams): 0 – Cholesterol (mg): 0 – Protein (grams): 15

   Dietary fiber (grams): 7 – Sodium (mg): 1,580 (much less if soup is homemade without

   salt and if bean spread is homemade with rinsed beans and no added salt)

   Calcium (mg): 117

Main Meal Menus
Menu One

- 1 cup lentil rice pilaf
- Baked sweet potato with 2 tsp. brown sugar and freshly squeezed lime juice
- 3/4 cup mixed, steamed greens with 2 tsp. slivered almonds
- Whole-grain corn muffin
- 1/2 cup fruit compote
- Water with lemon

  Calories: 592 – Fat (grams): 8 – Percent calories from fat: 12
  Saturated fat (grams): 1 – Cholesterol (mg): 21 (none, if muffin is homemade with egg substitute) – Protein (grams): 19 – Dietary fiber (grams): 14 – Sodium (mg): 269
  Iron (mg): 5 – Calcium (mg): 253

Menu Two

- 1 cup vegetable barley soup (low sodium)
- Spinach salad with sliced, ripe strawberries, 2 Tbsp. poppyseeds, and rice wine vinegar
- Homemade baked vegetable lasagna with soy cheese
- Sourdough roll
- 1 cup melon balls
- Water with lime

  Calories: 660 – Fat (grams): 16 – Percent calories from fat: 22
  Saturated fat (grams): 2 – Cholesterol (mg): 0 – Protein (grams): 28
  Dietary fiber (grams): 14 – Sodium (mg): 616 – Iron (mg): 9 – Calcium (mg): 547

Menu Three

- Mixed baby greens sprinkled with chopped walnuts and raspberry vinaigrette dressing
- 1 1/2 cups cooked linguine tossed with 1 cup steamed mixed vegetables, minced garlic, and 1 tsp. olive oil
- 4 pieces whole-grain flatbread
- Large piece of watermelon
- Water with lemon

  Calories: 541 – Fat (grams): 12 – Percent calories from fat: 20
  Saturated fat (grams): 1 – Cholesterol (mg): 0 – Protein (grams): 20
  Dietary fiber (grams): 16 – Sodium (mg): 286 – Iron (mg): 8 – Calcium (mg): 246

Menu Four
- 2 garbanzo-bean and rice-stuffed cabbage rolls on
- 1/2 cup stewed tomatoes with onions
- 1 cup boiled potatoes
- Thick chunk of multigrain bread
- Sliced kiwi
- Water with lemon

  Calories: 482 – Fat (grams): 3 – Percent calories from fat: 6

  Saturated fat (grams): 0 – Cholesterol (mg): 0 – Protein (grams): 12

  Dietary fiber (grams): 13 – Sodium (mg): 620 – Iron (mg): 4 – Calcium (mg): 148

Menu Five
- Black-bean burger on whole-grain bun with lettuce, tomato, and corn-salsa relish
- 1 cup spicy baked-potato wedges
- 3/4 cup steamed broccoli, cauliflower, and carrots
- Baked apple with brown sugar and cinnamon
- Hot herbal tea

  Calories: 487 – Fat (grams): 3 – Percent calories from fat: 6

  Saturated fat (grams): 0 – Cholesterol (mg): 0 – Protein (grams): 22

  Dietary fiber (grams): 15 – Sodium (mg): 581 – Iron (mg): 5 – Calcium (mg): 181

Menu Six
- 2 tofu-stuffed cannelloni with mushroom-marinara sauce
- 3/4 cup steamed, fresh green beans
- 3/4 cup roasted red potatoes
- Thick slice of Italian bread brushed with olive oil
- Clump of grapes
- Water with lemon

  Calories: 647 – Fat (grams): 11 – Percent calories from fat: 15

  Saturated fat (grams): 1 – Cholesterol (mg): 0 – Protein (grams): 20

  Dietary fiber (grams): 8 – Sodium (mg): 856 – Iron (mg): 5 – Calcium (mg): 176

Menu Seven

- Mixed green salad with orange and grapefruit sections and rice vinegar
- 3/4 cup curried chickpeas over
- 1 cup steamed jasmine rice
- 3/4 cup kale sauteed in 1 tsp. olive oil and minced garlic
- 2 peach halves
- Hot herbal tea

Calories: 581 – Fat (grams): 7 – Percent calories from fat: 11

Saturated fat (grams): 1 – Cholesterol (mg): 0 – Protein (grams): 20

Dietary fiber (grams): 10 – Sodium (mg): 69 – Iron (mg): 8 – Calcium (mg): 237

Sensible Snacks

Leftovers from lunch or dinner can be fine for a quick snack—grab some salad out of the refrigerator, or heat up a plate of yesterday's pasta in the microwave. What most snacks have in common is that they are quick. Some need to be portable and may need to fit into a purse, backpack, or briefcase. The sky's the limit, but here are some ideas to get you started:

- Flavored soy yogurt
- Instant soup with some whole-grain crackers
- Bran muffin
- Fresh seasonal fruit
- Low-fat popcorn
- Juice box
- Frozen fruit bar
- Bean burrito
- Bean taco
- Cinnamon-raisin bagel
- Low-fat oatmeal cookies
- Peeled baby carrots dipped in hummus or salsa
- Bowl of cereal
- Toast with jelly
- English muffin with apple butter
- Fresh fruit salad
- Vegetarian baked beans
- Baked potato topped with thick lentil soup
- Dried fruit (raisins, apricots, pears, apples, prunes)
- Frozen whole-grain waffle with applesauce
- Frozen banana
- Smoothie made with blenderized soymilk and fresh fruit

Recipe Modifications

Who needs recipes? Not me…not necessarily. Many of my favorite meals are the simplest ones to prepare—a big bowl of hot oatmeal with cinnamon and bits of fresh fruit; a baked sweet potato with a little brown sugar and fresh lime juice; or a plate of fettuccine tossed with a touch of olive oil, minced garlic, and chopped, fresh basil and topped with fresh diced tomatoes and a handful of pine nuts or a sprinkling of chopped walnuts.

I love to make my own wrap sandwiches with refried beans or hummus and chopped or shredded fresh vegetables, all rolled up together in a big, round piece of whole-grain lavash bread; I eat it burrito-style or cut into slices that look like pinwheels and are pretty on a plate. No recipes needed. These are strictly whip-it-up-fast dishes that are nevertheless delicious and nutritious.

I have a friend who maintains that recipes are fundamentally not necessary if you truly understand how to work with food. He feels that, rather than learning how to follow a recipe, people should instead, familiarize

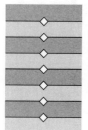

"It has been said (and probably by a good cook) that there are two kinds of people in the world: Those who are good cooks and those who wish they were good cooks. I hold that there is a third category: Those who are not good cooks and who couldn't care less. I am happily one of those."

—Helen Nearing, the late pioneering homesteader, in her book *Simple Food for the Good Life: An Alternative Cook Book* themselves with herbs and spices and learn how to judge which foods and flavors go best with which.

He believes that given practice, we could all become knowledgeable and confident enough to be able to take plain, unprocessed foods—grains, fruits, and vegetables—and combine them in pleasing ways, including flavoring them with herbs and spices, making use of whatever we have on hand at home or in the garden, or using whatever looks best at the supermarket or farmers' market. This, he rightly asserts, would result in wholesome meals from minimally processed foods prepared simply.

He likens this approach to the difference between learning about color theory and artistic composition and practicing painting vs. buying a kit for a paint-by-number picture. Although he didn't say it, he probably would also maintain that foods assembled creatively are more appealing, too, just as the artist's painting—no matter what the skill level—is more interesting and probably looks better than any paint-by-number picture could.

So although you don't need recipes to prepare meals, the material that follows does pertain to using recipes ... in the broad sense. The ideas for substitutions and for adding flavor without adding fat can be used to modify traditional recipes from your old Betty Crocker cookbook just as well as they can be used in your personal, no-recipe creations.

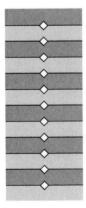

"Then I remembered a Frenchman and his wife who had eaten an extremely simple meal with us 20 years or so before, in our Vermont kitchen. The suave and elegant gentleman had enthused over a quickly thrown-together concoction. Wiping his lips, he said to his still more elegant wife, 'My dear, you must get the recipe of this delicious dish.' It was merely wheat berries, which he had never seen or tasted before, baked and sweetened with maple syrup and raisins. I could hardly have served them more simply, unless our guests had been asked to chew the wheat seed raw, which has also happened."

—Helen Nearing in *Simple Food for the Good Life*

Nifty Substitutions

I have memories of the television show Gilligan's Island, which I watched as a child when my mother permitted (she thought the show was "simple-minded" and usually encouraged me to turn it off). What still stands out most in my mind is how intrigued I was by how the ship-wrecked crew and passengers, marooned on that desert island, always seemed to have wonderful things to eat. I was especially mesmerized by the coconut cream and banana cream pies. Where did they get the milk, eggs, and butter they needed to make those pies? Okay, they used coconut milk in place of real milk, but what about the other ingredients? I was puzzled, captivated, and hungry.

I'm pleased to say, though, that I eventually solved that mystery. Did you know that milk, eggs, and butter aren't mandatory ingredients in such foods as cookies, pies, cakes, breads, and casseroles? In fact, there is a host of other ingredients that can take the place of those and serve the same functions—generally more healthfully, too. When I came to that realization, it was as if I'd struck gold. What freedom, and what possibilities!

Time Out

I had my own "island experience" a few years ago when I had a five-day layover in Fiji on a trip to Australia. I chose to stay on the little island of Beqa, just south of Fiji, at a tiny resort that was the only establishment on the island aside from the six small villages that dotted its shores. No stores, no T-shirt shops. Just thatched-roof bures, hammocks, and coconut palms.

A chef prepared the meals each day for the 12 or so guests, who all ate together, family style, in the open-air main bure. The chef shopped for groceries once a week on the main island and used fresh produce grown right on the premises or nearby. I told him I was a vegetarian and preferred to avoid animal products as much as possible. His response? "No problem." I was in for an incredible treat.

Breakfast typically consisted of an artfully-arranged plate of fresh papaya slices, slivers of melon, and chunks of fresh pineapple, which was picked nearby where it was growing wild in the bush. (It was here that I learned to squeeze fresh lime juice over my papaya slices for a sweet-tart flavor.) Fruit was followed by oatmeal pancakes with pure maple syrup, or freshly baked muffins.

The simple breakfasts were elegant, but there were a couple of lunch and dinner meals that stand out vividly in my memory because they were breathtakingly beautiful and they tasted so good, despite being made with absolutely no animal products.

One was a simple vegetable and pasta dish that was tossed with lots and lots of fresh basil. The aroma of fresh basil emanated from the kitchen from early morning all the way through lunchtime. Another day, while the other guests were eating fat- and cholesterol-laden cheese omelets, I feasted on an extraordinary vegetable-filled crepe. The tissue-thin crepe, made from rice flour, was folded over a bright assortment of lightly steamed, locally grown vegetables. The top of the crepe was garnished with some more colorful, grated vegetables and drizzled with a very clever "avocado cream." It was served with a refreshing mixed green salad with an herbed-vinegar dressing. The meal was a work of art.

One more meal stands out. A guide took me in a small boat to a deserted island one day and left me there alone for the day with just my snorkeling gear, a straw mat, and a huge cooler packed with my lunch and snacks. As soon as the guide's boat disappeared from sight, I peeked inside the cooler.

Inside, I found a large bottle of mineral water, a gorgeous plated arrangement of tropical fruits, a big bowl of cold pasta salad, and chunks of fresh sourdough bread. If you disregard the Coke and the Hershey bar, it was another example of a beautiful, healthful and satisfying meal created without animal products.

Back to Reality

Isn't it funny, though—strange, in a way. Open your Betty Crocker or Fannie Farmer cookbook, your *Joy of Cooking* or your Better Homes, and what do you notice about most of the recipes? Almost every one includes animal products. If a cookie or cake recipe exists that doesn't call for milk, butter, and eggs, I haven't found it. Our cookbooks reflect our culture. We are a culture that gives animal products a central role in our diets. They are incorporated into almost everything we eat.

I'm older and wiser now, and I have worked all of the milk, eggs, and but-

ter out of my culinary repertoire. I enjoy using the substitutions that follow—the foods taste great, and I feel good knowing that the ingredients
are more healthful. I also take special pleasure in knowing that, even if
marooned on a desert island without an egg in sight, I'd still be able to
make my favorite foods.

Replacements for Eggs
In Baked Goods ...

Eggs function as binders and leavening agents in baked
goods and can easily be replaced and, sometimes, even left out of recipes
without significantly affecting the flavor or texture of the product. For
instance, in foods that do not require a great deal of leavening, such as
cookies and pancakes, the eggs can be left out altogether if the recipe calls
for only one or two eggs. Add a tablespoon or two of additional liquid to
the batter to maintain the intended moisture content, and the food should
turn out fine.

On the other hand, if you do want to replace the eggs in a baked good
recipe with something that will add lightness to the product, try one of the
following substitutions:

Instead of one whole egg, use:

- 1/2 of a small, ripe banana, mashed. This will add a banana flavor
  to the food item, so use it in foods in which you don't mind that
  flavor, such as in muffins, cookies, and pancakes.
- 1/4 cup applesauce, canned pumpkin, or pureed prunes. Like the
  bananas, these may also add a bit of flavor to the food. When you
  use mashed fruits to replace eggs, the result is often a denser
  baked good, since fruit doesn't add leavening power to the recipe.
  If you would prefer to lighten the recipe, you can add an extra half
  teaspoon of baking powder.
- 1/4 cup tofu blended with the liquid ingredients in the recipe. You
  can use "light" tofu to reduce the fat and calories in the product.
- 1 1/2 tsp. of Ener-G Egg Replacer mixed with 2 Tbsp. of water. This
  is one of my favorite egg substitutes—it's convenient and works
  very well in baked goods. You'll find it in natural foods stores and
  in some supermarkets. It is a powder made from vegetable
  starches.

- A heaping tablespoon of soy flour or bean flour mixed with 1 Tbsp. of water
- 2 Tbsp. of cornstarch beaten with 2 Tbsp. of water
- 1 Tbsp. of finely ground flax seeds whipped with 1/4 cup of water

In Burgers, Loaves, and Casseroles ...

When eggs are used in recipes for casseroles, patties, and meatloaf-type foods, their function is as a binder to hold the food together. For these substitutions, you may need to experiment with the amount of the replacer to use, but you can generally start out by using 2 or 3 table-spoons to replace one egg. Also, keep this in mind as you consider the substitutions that follow. Some of these egg replacers will affect the flavor of the food. Try the following:

- Mashed potatoes, mashed sweet potatoes, or instant potato flakes
- Quick-cooking rolled oats or cooked oatmeal
- Fine bread crumbs, cracker meal, or matzo meal
- Flour—whole wheat, unbleached white, oat
- Arrowroot starch, potato starch, cornstarch, or Ener-G Egg Replacer
- Tomato paste
- 1/4 cup tofu blended with 1 Tbsp. of flour

In Other Recipes ...

Did you know that tofu makes a wonderful substitute for chopped eggs in salads and sandwiches? Add cubes of tofu to green salads instead of using eggs; marinate the tofu cubes in your favorite dressing to add flavor. You can also substitute mashed or chopped tofu for the eggs in traditional egg salad sandwich recipes. Another idea: Use tofu instead of eggs to make "scrambled tofu." Many vegetarian or soy cookbooks give recipes for this, or you can buy a "tofu scrambler" spice mix at most natural-foods stores and in some supermarkets. Scrambled tofu is great for breakfast or as a sandwich filling in pita pockets or in a Kaiser roll.

Replacements for Milk and Other Dairy Products

To replace milk... This one is very easy! There are numerous nondairy beverage products on the market now that can be used cup for cup to replace cow's milk in recipes or on breakfast cereal. My favorite is soymilk, because it generally is the most nutritious choice. I buy the fortified variety for the extra vitamin D, vitamin B12, and calcium it contains.

Soymilk has a slight "beany" aftertaste that I find very pleasant. Plain soymilk is a good substitute for cow's milk in savory recipes. I buy vanilla-flavored soymilk to use on my cereal and for sweeter recipes such as desserts or fruit smoothies that I make in the blender.

Nondairy milk replacers can be found in almost every supermarket now, but the biggest selection is still likely to be found at a natural foods store. Although you may find some soymilk in powdered form or refrigerated in the dairy case, most nondairy beverages are now packaged in aseptic cartons—the kind that don't need refrigeration until they are opened. In addition to soymilk, you'll see rice milk, potato milk, oat milk, almond milk, and rice and soy blends.

There is a lot of variation in flavor among all of these products, so you may need to try several before settling on your favorite. Most are available in plain, vanilla, and carob flavors, as well. The nutritional compositions vary from brand to brand, so read the labels carefully. My personal favorite is Edensoy Plus, vanilla-flavored. At the natural foods store where I buy mine, there is a 10% discount when I buy a case.

You can make your own buttermilk substitute for recipes by adding 2 tsp. of lemon juice or vinegar to one cup of whichever milk replacer you use.

To replace cheese... There are many soy- and nut-based cheese substitutes on the market that can be found in natural foods stores. Although they are cholesterol-free and low in saturated fat, many do contain a fair amount of vegetable fat. They are best in recipes in which they are one of several ingredients as opposed to being eaten alone (or with fruit or crackers). For example, soy cheese is good mixed into casseroles, and the mozzarella-style is good on pizza.

Soy-based Parmesan cheese substitute is available, but nutritional yeast, found in natural foods stores, also works well as a "cheesy-tasting" condiment sprinkled over pasta or popcorn.

Tofu mashed with a few teaspoons of lemon juice can be substituted for ricotta cheese or cottage cheese in recipes such as lasagna or stuffed shells.

To replace yogurt and sour cream... Flavored soy yogurts are delicious; use the plain variety to replace regular yogurt or sour cream in dips and sauces.

To replace butter... Soy margarine can be used instead of butter, as can other forms of margarine. The key to choosing the best butter substitute is to find a product with the least amount of saturated fat. Aim for a margarine with not more than one gram of saturated fat per serving.

You can also use about 7/8 of a cup of vegetable oil to replace one cup of butter in recipes, although this substitution won't work in all baked goods. To reduce the amount of total fat in recipes, see Adding Flavor Without Fat on page 182.

Replacements for Meat

There are many creative ways to replace the meat in recipes with vegetable- or grain-based ingredients, and by doing so, you'll eliminate the cholesterol and markedly reduce the saturated fat content of your meal. Try some of these ideas for starters:

Use textured vegetable protein (TVP) to replace the ground meat in tacos, burritos, sloppy Joe sauce, and chili. It works beautifully in these products; you'll love it. You can find it at natural foods stores in dried form in boxes or in bulk bins, and many supermarkets now carry a similar product in the frozen foods section.

Bulgur wheat (rolled, cracked wheat) can also be used to add a ground beef-like texture to chili. Make bean chili and toss in a handful of bulgur wheat for texture.

Experiment with recipes using tofu, tempeh, and seitan. Tofu, which is soybean curd that has been pressed into a block, can be cut into cubes and stir-fried; the firm style can withstand being jostled around without falling apart. You can also freeze tofu. Once thawed, it has a chewier, more meaty texture.

Tempeh is a soy product made from whole soybeans. It's sold in block-like pieces that are about a half-inch think, and it can be used in many of the same ways that meat is used—barbecued, used in chunks in stews or with sauces, in strips in sandwiches, and so on.

Seitan (pronounced Say'tan) is a chewy product made from wheat gluten, or wheat protein, that is also versatile as a meat substitute. You can often find seitan, or gluten, dishes on the menus at Chinese or Thai restaurants. You'll find tofu dishes on the menus, too. It can be fun to try these foods at a restaurant first, before cooking with them yourself, to familiarize yourself with how they can taste when they are prepared in traditional ways.

Vegetarian hot dogs are available in natural foods stores and in many supermarkets, and they are a delicious substitute for the "real" thing. Cholesterol-free, they are also free of or very low in saturated fat and are generally lower in sodium and higher in protein than meat hot dogs. They're good in beans-n-franks, and are a great idea for picnics, cookouts, or to have on hand for teens who want a quick meal. Also try vegetarian bacon and sausage substitutes; they work well in recipes that call for the meat varieties.

Vegetarian burger patties come in many varieties and can be found in most supermarkets and in all-natural foods stores. Like vegetarian hot dogs, vegetarian burger patties are far superior nutritionally to meat burgers. They can be used "as is" or can be crumbled to use in recipes such as sloppy Joes or in taco and burrito fillings.

Beans have been a staple food throughout the world for thousands of years. They are extremely versatile and can be used as the basis for many hearty dishes in place of meat. Bean chili can be made with kidney beans, chili beans, or a mixture of several different types of beans. A handful of corn adds even more color. In addition to bean chili, bean burritos, bean tacos, bean soups, bean stews, and bean casseroles are a great place to start using beans in place of meat.

Dried beans can be soaked overnight, then cooked, or they can be cooked in a pressure cooker. If you are inclined to use a pressure cooker, a terrific cookbook is *Great Vegetarian Cooking Under Pressure* by Lorna Sass, Morrow, New York, N.Y., 1994. Canned beans are also a perfectly acceptable alternative to dried beans. To reduce the sodium content of canned beans, rinse them with water before using them. You can also find dehydrated bean flakes in the natural foods store. They are super-convenient for making burrito and taco fillings as well as bean dips. I buy the black bean and the pinto bean varieties.

Adding Flavor Without Adding Fat

Fat serves several purposes in recipes. It can help to marry other flavors in the recipe and to carry the flavor throughout the dish. It can add a flavor of its own to foods and can also add moisture and texture to baked goods.

Unfortunately, fat packs a great many calories and when fat comes from animal sources, it creates health problems. While it may not be necessary to eliminate every speck of fat from recipes, many recipes are so high in fat that some degree of modification can create a product that is more healthful and substantially lower in calories.

I have one product in mind that is a good example. My favorite neighborhood supermarket has its own bakery and is known for its delicious muffins. One sad day, however, the local newspaper printed the fat content of those muffins, a figure that had not previously been available to customers. The terrible news: one muffin contained 30 grams of fat—far too much fat by anyone's standards, particularly when so many people I knew were eating at least one muffin per day, sometimes two.

The culprit in those muffins was the oil. Many muffin recipes call for at least one cup of oil per batch. If you make your own muffins instead, you can substantially reduce the amount of oil you add to the batter without sacrificing too much in the way of texture or flavor.

Fat can often be reduced in recipes without mortally wounding the final product. On the other hand, some recipes in which the fat has been lowered do result in a product that has a different flavor or texture than the original recipe intended. It depends on the product and how much the recipe has been altered.

I've made quick breads and muffins in which I have substituted applesauce for much of the fat in the recipe, and the result has been a denser, chewier, spongier bread or muffin. If my product were being graded in a traditional cooking school, I would probably be marked down for those qualities. However, I happen to find those qualities appealing—it doesn't bother me that my muffins have a different texture. So when you modify a recipe to lower its fat content, realize that, while some qualities of the product may change (especially texture, I have found), you may not find those changes diminish your enjoyment of that product.

Here are some ways to replace fat in recipes:

Invest in some good nonstick pots and pans, and eliminate or cut down on the amount of fat that you add when you saute vegetables. For instance, when I fix steamed kale, I put a drop of olive oil on the bottom of a skillet—just enough to keep the minced garlic, which I add next, from sticking. Then I add about 1/4 inch of water or vegetable stock to the pan, bring it to a simmer, and add the kale. I cover the skillet and steam the kale, stirring occasionally, for a few minutes until the kale is soft.

You can also add wine or cooking sherry to the pan when you saute vegetables. The key is to keep the oil to a minimum and to add another flavorful liquid to "saute/steam" or "stir/steam" the vegetables.

You can usually reduce the amount of fat called for in recipes for baked goods by a least one-third without adversely affecting the outcome. For instance, if a cookie recipe calls for one cup of butter, you can probably reduce that to 2/3 cup (and use a low-saturated fat margarine instead of butter) without noticing any difference in the quality of the cookies.

As I noted earlier, the difference you are most likely to see when you reduce the fat in baked goods is a denser and chewier texture. Sometimes, though, reducing the fat in a recipe will make the end product dry. I've reduced the fat in some cookie recipes and ended up with little rocks instead of chewy, soft cookies. You'll have to experiment to see what works. Hint: Keep notes of the changes that you make when you modify recipes, so that if you find a substitution that works wonderfully, you'll be able to duplicate your creation!

Substitute mashed fruit for some or all of the fat in recipes. Replacing half of the fat in a recipe with fruit will probably work well. If you replace more fat than that, you'll need to experiment to see what you can get away with. You can try applesauce, pureed prunes, pumpkin (okay, it's a vegetable), mashed banana, or combinations of one of more of these. If you use banana, remember that your product will take on a banana flavor (which can taste great!).

If recipes call for nuts, cut back on the amount you use to reduce fat and calories. In some recipes, other foods can substitute for the crunch that nuts add. For example, minced water chestnuts can add crunch to salads, side dishes, and casseroles that call for nuts, and Grapenuts cereal or fat-free granola can add an crunchy texture to baked goods that call for nuts.

You can make cream soups without using whole milk or cream by pureeing potato with vegetable broth and mixing it into the soup or by using pureed soft tofu in the same way. I've had soups at vegetarian restaurants that I swore were made with cream, only to be shocked to learn that they were dairy-free. It works. You can make bean, pea, and lentil soups creamy by pureeing part of the soup and mixing the pureed portion back into the rest of the soup.

Experiment with herbs and spices to add flavor to foods. A squeeze of fresh lemon juice or a dash of seasoned rice vinegar or hot sauce can add lots of zip to vegetables without adding fat. Fresh herbs have a great deal more flavor than the dried variety, so consider planting an herb garden at home. Even a small window garden will work. Once you begin using fresh herbs, you'll be hooked.

Recommended Dietary Allowances
and Dietary Reference Intakes

———————————————◇———————————————

The following Recommended Dietary Allowances, expressed as average daily intakes over time, were established by the Food and Nutrition Board, National Academy of Sciences. The recommendations are designed for the maintenance of good nutrition for practically all healthy people in the United States. As always, the best eating style is based on adequate calories and a variety of foods. That way, you'll be sure to get the required nutrients, even those for which requirements have been less well defined.

Recommended Dietary Allowances

	Age	Protein (G)	Vitamins A (MCG RE)	E (MG)	K (MCG)	C (MG)
INFANTS	0-6 mos	13	375	3	5	30
	6-12 mos	14	375	4	10	35
CHILDREN	1-3 yrs	16	400	6	15	40
	4-6	24	500	7	20	45
	7-10	28	700	7	30	45
MALES	11-14 yrs	45	1000	10	45	50
	15-18	59	1000	10	65	60
	19-24	58	1000	10	70	60
	25-50	63	1000	10	80	60
	51+	63	1000	10	80	60
FEMALES	11-14 yrs	46	800	8	45	50
	15-18	44	800	8	55	60
	19-24	46	800	8	60	60
	25-50	50	800	8	65	60
	51+	50	800	8	65	60
PREGNANT		60	800	10	65	70
LACTATING	1st 6 mos	65	1300	12	65	95
	2nd 6 mos	62	1200	11	65	90

Recommended Dietary Allowances

| | | MINERALS | | | |
	AGE	IRON (MG)	ZINC (MG)	IODINE (MCG)	SELENIUM (MCG)
INFANTS	0-6 mos	6	5	40	10
	6-12 mos	10	5	50	15
CHILDREN	1-3 yrs	10	10	70	20
	4-6	10	10	90	20
	7-10	10	10	120	30
MALES	11-14 yrs	12	15	150	40
	15-18	12	15	150	50
	19-24	10	15	150	70
	25-50	10	15	150	70
	51+	10	15	150	70
FEMALES	11-14 yrs	15	12	150	45
	15-18	15	12	150	50
	19-24	15	12	150	55
	25-50	15	12	150	55
	51+	10	12	150	55
PREGNANT		30	15	175	65
LACTATING	1st 6 mos	15	19	200	75
	2nd 6 mos	15	16	200	75

Adapted with permission from Recommended Dietary Allowances, 10th Edition.
© 1989 *by the National Academy of Sciences. Published by National Academy Press, Washington, DC.*

mcg RE = *microgram Retinol Equivalents*
mcg = *micrograms*
mg = *milligrams*
g = *grams*

Dietary Reference Intakes (DRIs)

Age/ Life–Stage	Calcium (mg)	Phosphorus (mg)	Magnesium (mg)	Vitamin D[a, b] (mcg)	Flouride (mg)	Thiamin (mg)
INFANTS						
0–5 months	210*	100*	30*	5*	0.01*	0.2*
6–11 months	270*	275*	75*	5*	0.5*	0.3*
CHILDREN						
1–3 yrs .	500*	460	80	5*	0.7*	0.5
4–8 yrs.	800*	500	130	5*	1*	0.6
MALES						
9–13 yrs.	1300*	1250	240	5*	2*	0.9
14–18 yrs.	1300*	1250	410	5*	3*	1.2
19–30 yrs.	1000*	700	400	5*	4*	1.2
31–50 yrs.	1000*	700	420	5*	4*	1.2
51–70 yrs.	1200*	700	420	10*	4*	1.2
>70 yrs.	1200*	700	420	15*	4*	1.2
FEMALES						
9–13 yrs.	1300*	1250	240	5*	2*	0.9
14–18 yrs.	1300*	1250	360	5*	3*	1.0
19–30 yrs.	1000*	700	310	5*	3*	1.1
31–50 yrs.	1000*	700	320	5*	3*	1.1
51–70 yrs.	1200*	700	320	10*	3*	1.1
>70 yrs.	1200*	700	320	15*	3*	1.1
PREGNANCY						
≤ 18 yrs.	1300*	1250	400	5*	3*	1.4
19–30 yrs.	1000*	700	350	5*	3*	1.4
31–50 yrs.	1000*	700	360	5*	3*	1.4
LACTATION						
≤ 18 yrs.	1300*	1250	360	5*	3*	1.5
19–30 yrs.	1000*	700	310	5*	3*	1.5
31–50 yrs.	1000*	700	320	5*	3*	1.5

mg = milligrams   ; mcg = micrograms

*Note: This table presents Recommended Dietary Allowances (RDAs) and Adequate Intakes (AIs). (AI values are followed by an asterisk.) RDAs and AIs may both be used as goals for individual intake. RDAs are set to meet the average daily needs of almost all (97 to 98 per-

Riboflavin (mg)	Niacin[c] (mg)	Vitamin B$_6$ (mg)	Folate[d] (mcg)	Vitamin B$_{12}$ (mcg)	Pantothenic Acid (mg)	Biotin (mcg)	Choline[e] (mg)
0.3*	2*	0.1*	65*	0.4*	1.7*	5*	125*
0.4*	3*	0.3*	80*	0.5*	1.8*	6*	150*
0.5	6	0.5	150	0.9	2*	8*	200*
0.6	8	0.6	200	1.2	3*	12*	250*
0.9	12	1.0	300	1.8	4*	20*	375*
1.3	16	1.3	400	2.4	5*	25*	550*
1.3	16	1.3	400	2.4	5*	30*	550*
1.3	16	1.3	400	2.4	5*	30*	550*
1.3	16	1.7	400	2.4[f]	5*	30*	550*
1.3	16	1.7	400	2.4[f]	5*	30*	550*
0.9	12	1.0	300	1.8	4*	20*	375*
1.0	14	1.2	400[g]	2.4	5*	25*	400*
1.1	14	1.3	400[g]	2.4	5*	30*	425*
1.1	14	1.3	400[g]	2.4	5*	30*	425*
1.1	14	1.5	400[g]	2.4[f]	5*	30*	425*
1.1	14	1.5	400	2.4[f]	5*	30*	425*
1.4	18	1.9	600[h]	2.6	6*	30*	450*
1.4	18	1.9	600[h]	2.6	6*	30*	450*
1.4	18	1.9	600[h]	2.6	6*	30*	450*
1.6	17	2.0	500	2.8	7*	35*	550*
1.6	17	2.0	500	2.8	7*	35*	550*
1.6	17	2.0	500	2.8	7*	35*	550*

see notes on next page

cent) healthy individuals in a life-stage group. The AIs are believed to cover the daily needs of most healthy people, but lack of data or uncertainty in the data prevent clear specification of an RDA.

Notes to "Dietary Reference Intakes (DRIs)," (page 189)

[a] As cholecalciferol (1mcg cholecalciferol = 40 IU vitamin D)

[b] In the absence of adequate exposure to sunlight.

[c] As niacin equivalents. 1mg of niacin = 60 mg of tryptophan

[d] As dietary folate equivalents (DFE). 1 DFE = 1 mcg food folate = 0.6 mcg of folic acid (from fortified food or supplement) consumed with food = 0.5 mcg of supplemental folic acid taken on an empty stomach.

[e] Although AIs have been set for choline, there are few data to assess whether a dietary supply of choline is needed at all stages of the life cycle.

[f] Since 10 to 30 percent of older people may malabsorb food–bound B_{12}, it is advisable for those older than 50 yrs. to meet their RDA mainly by taking foods fortified with B_{12} or a B_{12} containing supplement.

[g] It is recommended that all women capable of becoming pregnant consume 400 mcg of folic acid from fortified foods and/or supplements in addition to intake of food folate from a varied diet.

[h] Women should continue taking 400 mcg of folic acid until their pregnancy is confirmed, at which time the recommended daily intake increases.

Chart adapted with permission from the National Academy of Sciences. Copyright 1997 and 1998.

Index

A

additives, 75
airplane travel
  airline lounges and clubs, 138–139
  beverage service, 142
  cafeterias, 137–138
  check real hunger, 142–143
  food stands, 135–137
  in-flight meals, 139–140
  newsstands, 135
  peanuts, 142
  restaurants, 138
  special meals, 140–141
  vegan meals, 140
alcohol, 139, 155
American Cancer Society
  dietary guidelines, 8
American Dietetic Association (ADA)
  address for, 146
  difficulty in moving away from, 17–19
  food industries and financial support
    of, 10–12, 15
  promoting plant-based diets, 22
  referral service of, 49, 84, 146
  web site for, 150
animal foods
  environmental contaminants in, 78
  in optimal diet, 83
aspartame, 73

B

balanced diet concept
  traditional American diet and, 9
  vagueness of, 15–17
beans
  as calcium source, 34
  meal-planning guide, 158–160
  as meat substitute, 181
  versatility of, 103
beta carotene, 26

blood sugar levels
  fiber and, 53
books
  about plant-based diets, 147–149
  cookbooks, 148–149
breads
  meal-planning guide, 156–157
brown bag take-along food, 132–133
butter
  replacement for, 180

C

calcium
  children's needs for, 32–34
  green, leafy vegetables as source of,
    29–30
  milk as source of, 29–30
  phosphates and, 11, 31
  plant-based sources of, 34–35
  protein consumption and, 9, 30–31
  recommended dietary allowance of,
    9
  sodium and, 31, 75
  Vitamin D, 31–32
candy
  best choices of, 135
canned goods
  starter staples for, 104
carcinogens
  saccharin as, 73–74
Center for Science in the Public
  Interest, 146
  web site for, 150
cereals
  meal-planning guide, 156–157
cheese
  replacements for, 179–180
cheese-and-egg rut, 84–85, 95

children
  adventurous spirit in trying new
    foods, 98
  books on plant-based diets for, 148
  calcium needs of, 32–34
  cookbooks for, 149
  fat needs for, 50, 84, 95
  food jags and, 99
  giving choices, 98
  growing vegetables, 99
  helping with shopping, 98
  low-fat plant-based diet for, 95,
    97–99
  physical activity for, 50
  preparing meals, 99
  school meals system and, 99–100
  setting good examples for, 99
  snacks for, 95
  weight control for, 50
Chinese restaurant tips, 144
cholesterol
  fiber and, 53
coffee
  gourmet coffee stands, 136–137
  iron absorption and, 36
colon cancer
  fiber and, 53
condiments
  starter staples for, 105
  sugar and salt in, 79
constipation
  fiber and, 52–53
cookbooks, 148–149
cooler take-along food, 132–133
couscous, 157

D
daidzein, 54
dairy industry
  dietary guidelines and, 5–6
dairy products
  Asian population and, 30
  children's needs for, 32
  decreasing amount to increase veg-
    etables, fruit and grains, 54–55
  egg replacements, 177–178
  fat in, 45
  lack of fiber in, 27–28
  as primary sources of saturated fat
    and cholesterol, 27

  protein consumption and, 28–29
  replacements for, 179–180
  requirements for, 28–29, 29–30
  variety of food concept, 25–27,
    27–28, 39
Derelian, Doris, 10, 12, 15
diet
  balanced diet concept, 9
  traditional American, 9
dietary continuum, 84–86
  changing, 85–86
dietary guidelines
  basing on scientific information,
    19–20
  consumer's need for straightforward
    advice, 5–7
  food industries and health organiza-
    tion's politics, 5–7
  lack of specificity in, 7, 9, 13
Dietary Guidelines Alliance
  members of, 7
Dietary Reference Intakes, 188–190
dietitian
  help from, 49, 84, 146
dry items
  starter staples for, 104

E
eating out, 109–121
  atmosphere, 111–112
  avoiding mass-produced food, 112
  baked potatoes, 111
  pasta, 111
  restaurant owners/chefs' tips,
    112–121
  side dishes, 111
  substitutions for potato chips/fries,
    111
  tips for different types of, 143–144
  tips for different types of restaurants,
    143–144
eggs
  replacements for, 177–178
entertaining. *See* social situations
environmental contaminants
  in animal products, 78
  fiber and, 78
  in plants, 78
Equal, 73
ethnic grocery stores, 102

exercise. *See* physical activity

F

fast-food restaurant tips, 143
fat
  5% of calories, 61
  10% of calories, 19–20, 64, 68
  15–20% of calories, 68
  30% of calories, 19–20, 64
  adults need for, 95
  bodies need for, 61
  calories in, 44
  children's need for, 50, 95
  in dairy products, 45
  decrease of, and increase in fiber, 44
  eating less meats and dairy products
    to reduce, 63
  fat-free substitutes and, 65
  grains, fruits and vegetables instead
    of meat/dairy, 67
  in grains and vegetables, 61–62
  heart disease reversal program and,
    64, 68, 70
  limiting to 30% vs. 10%, 19–20
  in meat, 45
  recipe modification to reduce,
    182–184
  recommendations in grams per day,
    68–69
  saturated, 70
  in traditional American diet, 44
  type of and total fat, 66
  weight control and 15–20% of calo-
    ries for, 68
fat-free substitutes, 65
fiber
  blood sugar levels and, 53
  cholesterol-lowering effect of, 5, 53
  colon cancer and, 53
  constipation and, 52–53
  content in grams of common foods,
    58–59
  decrease in fat, and increase in, 44
  environmental contaminants and, 78
  flatulence and increase in, 58
  grains, vegetables and fruits as
    source of, 52–54
  recommendations for, 27
  supplements, 54
  30 gram/day goal, 57, 69

  typical American consumption of, 27
  water and, 59
5 a Day campaign, 51
flatulence
  fiber increase and, 58
food co-ops, 151
food groups
  daily serving sizes for meal-planning,
    154–155
  vs. plant foods and animal foods,
    37–38
Food Guide Pyramid, 51–52
food industries
  financial support of ADA, 10–12, 15
Food Marketing Institute, 7
food stands
  at airports, 135–137
freezer
  starter staples for, 105
frozen yogurt, 135–136
fruits
  5 a Day campaign, 51
  in Food Guide Pyramid, 51–52
  less animal products for more, 54–55
  meal-planning guide, 160–161
  phytochemicals in, 54
  pre-wash and pre-cut, 106
  as source of fiber, 52–54

G

genistein, 54
government health organizations
  economic pressure on, 6–8
  politics of dietary guidelines, 6–8
grains
  fat in, 61–62
  in Food Guide Pyramid, 51–52
  less animal products for more, 54–55
  phytochemicals in, 54
  as source of fiber, 52–54
Great Vegetarian Cooking Under Pressure
  (Sass), 181

H

hard in and soft out, 53
Health and Human Services (HHS)
  Dietary Guidelines, 6
heart disease reversal program, 19–20,
  64, 68, 70

high-protein plant products
  meal-planning guide, 158–160
home, making diet changes, 93–107
  children and, 97–99
  cupboard, fridge, and freezer staples,
    103–105
  discord from divergent food habits,
    93–96
  every adult responsible for self,
    96–97
  importance of support of everyone,
    93–94
  planning ahead, 106
  setting an example, 96, 97, 99
  stocking your kitchen, 101–102
  time-saving tips, 106–107

I

Indian restaurant tips, 144
International Food Information
  Council, 7
iron
  coffee and teas, 36
  sources of, 36
isoflavonoids, 54
Italian restaurant tips, 143

J

junk food, 83

L

lactose intolerance, 30, 31
  ethnic groups and, 30, 31
legumes. See beans
low-fat foods
  as bulky and filling, 44
  fiber and, 44
  recipe modification for, 182–184

M

magazines
  about plant-based diets, 150
mannitol, 73
meal-planning guide, 153–161
  breads, 156–157
  cereals, 156–157
  food group daily servings sizes,
    154–155
  fruits, 160–161

legumes and high-protein plant
  products, 158–160
  vegetables, 157–158
meat
  decreasing amount to increase veg-
    etables, fruit and grains, 54–55
  eating less and effect on calcium,
    30–31
  fat in, 45
  lack of fiber in, 27–28
  moving away from diet centered on,
    17–19
  politics of guidelines for, 8
  as primary sources of saturated fat
    and cholesterol, 27
  replacements for, 180–181
  variety of food concept, 25–27,
    27–28, 39
meat industry
  Dietary Guidelines and, 5–6
menus, 163–171
  breakfast, 163–166
  light meals, 166–168
  main meals, 169–171
  sensible snacks, 172
Mexican restaurant tips, 144
milk. See also dairy products
  replacements for, 179–180
moderation concept
  vagueness of, 15–17

N

National Cattlemen's Beef Association,
  7
National Center for Nutrition and
  Dietetics, 10–11, 146
National Dairy Council, 5–6, 7
National Food Processors Association,
  7
National Pork Producers Council, 7
New Century Garden Guide, 37–40
  variety of foods in, 38–39
newsletters
  about plant-based diets, 150
newsstands
  at airports, 135
no good or bad food concept, 12,
  13–15
Nutrasweet, 73

Nutrient Standard Menu Planning,
    100–101
nutrition
    big-picture approach to, 5
nuts, 26, 136, 142, 160

O

optimal diet
    animal foods as side dish in, 83
    calories in, 83
    fat in, 83–84
    foods as close to natural state as
        possible, 84
    outside our culture, 89–91
    salt in, 83–84
    variety in, 83
organics
    advantages of, 75
    expense of, 75, 77
osteoporosis
    defined, 32
    lifestyle factors for, 32

P

pasta, 156
    at restaurants, 111
peanuts, 26, 142, 160
pesticides, 75
phosphates
    calcium, 31
physical activity
    amount of, 43
    controlling weight and, 42
    increasing, to increase calorie intake,
        42, 46–47, 83
    kid's need for, 50
    list of activities for fun and fitness, 48
    moderate to vigorous physical daily,
        47–48
Physicians Committee for Responsible
    Medicine, 146
phytochemicals
    defined, 54
phytoestrogens, 54
pizza shop tips, 144
plant-based diet, 18. See also optimal
    diet
    books about, 147–149
    cheese-and-egg rut, 84–85
    large variety available for, 38–39

low-fat diet for children, 95
magazines and newsletters, 150
New Century Garden Guide, 37–40
vitamin B12, 38
plant-to-animal products ratio, 56–57
politics
    defined, 5
    putting into perspective, 20–23
popcorn
    sold at stands, 137
potassium chloride, 74–75
preservatives, 75
pretzels, soft, 135
Produce Marketing Association, 7
protein
    calcium needs and, 9, 28–29, 30–31
    meat vs. bean choice, 28–29
    plant sources of, 35–36

R

recipe modification, 173–184
    adding flavor without fat, 182–184
    egg replacements, 177–178
    meat replacement, 180–181
    milk/dairy products replacements,
        179–180
Recommended Dietary Allowances,
    186–187
refrigerator
    starter staples for, 105
restaurant tips, 109–121. See also eating
    out
    atmosphere, 111–112
    avoiding mass-produced food, 112
    baked potatoes, 111
    Chinese, 144
    fast-food, 143–144
    Indian, 144
    Italian, 143
    Mexican, 144
    pasta, 111
    pizza shops, 144
    restaurant owners/chefs' tips,
        112–121
    side dishes, 111
    substitutions for potato chips/fries,
        111
    tips for different types of, 143–144
rice, 156
    making extra, 107

S

saccharin, 73
  as carcinogen, 73–74
salads
  making extra big, 106–107
salt
  calcium and, 31
  common ways people add to diet, 74
  in condiments, 79
  limiting, 79
  negative effect of, 75
  in optimal diet, 83–84
  taste for, 74
salt substitutes, 74, 80
school meals system
  changes in, 100
  guidelines for, 20–21
  Nutrient Standard Menu Planning,
    100–101
seitan, 181
shopping
  from a list, 102
  style of, 102–103
Shopping for Health: A Nutritionist's Aisle-
  By-Aisle Guide to Smart, Low Fat Choices
  at the Supermarket (Havala), 79, 104
Simple, Lowfat & Vegetarian (Havala), 112
snacks
  for children, 95
  cooler and brown bag take-alongs,
    132–133
  good choices for, 49
  sensible, 172
  starter staples for, 104
social situations, 123–130
  anticipate complications, 125
  be assertive, 126–127
  breaking from family tradition,
    123–124
  broken record technique, 126
  don't preach, 127
  educate and inform others, 125–126
  as guest, 128–129
  as host, 129–130
  orient social events to activities
    rather than food, 127
sodium. *See also* salt
  calcium and, 31

common ways people add to diet, 74
  negative effect of, 75
soft drinks, 83
  calcium and, 31
  phosphates in, and calcium, 11
soft in and hard out, 53
sorbitol, 73
sour cream
  replacement for, 180
soy foods, 159
  as dairy product replacements,
    179–180
Soy of Cooking (Oser), 159
soyfood
  as meat replacement, 180–181
soymilk, 31, 159, 179
Sprinkle Sweet, 73
staples
  starter staples for cupboard, fridge
    and freezers, 103–105
sugar, 72
  in condiments, 79
  as empty calories, 72
  limiting, 79
  in optimal diet, 83–84
  types of, 72
Sugar Association, 7
sugar substitutes, 73–74, 80
Sugar Twin, 73
support
  advocate for yourself, 151
  books about plant-based diets,
    147–149
  community, 151
  food co-ops, 151
  local vegetarian societies, 151
  magazines and newsletters, 150
  organizations for, 146–147
  other materials, 150
  self-help/nutrition education,
    145–146
  web sites for, 150
Sweet N' Low, 73

T

tea
  iron absorption and, 36
tempeh, 180–181
textured vegetable protein, 180
tofu, 159, 177, 178, 180

Tofu Cookery (Hagler), 159
traditional American diet
    balanced diet concept and, 9
    culture of, 89–91
    fat in, 44
    first steps in moving away from, 86
    optimal diet vs., 82–83
trail mix, 136
traveling eating advise, 131–144
    by airplane, 134–143
    in the car, 132–133
    cooler and brown bag take-alongs,
        132–133
    on cruises, 133–134
    restaurant tips for, 143–144

U

United States Department of
    Agriculture (USDA) Dietary
    Guidelines, 6
    school lunch program and, 20–21

V

variety of food concept
    dairy products and, 25–27, 39
    diluting negative consequences of
        single food, 25–26
    meats and, 25–27, 39
    in optimal diet, 83
    for plant-based diet, 36–37
    plant world's large variety, 39
    vagueness of, 15–17
vegan meals, 140
vegetables
    fat in, 61–62
    5 a Day campaign, 51
    in Food Guide Pyramid, 51–52
    less animal products for more, 54–55
    meal-planning guide, 157–158
    phytochemicals in, 54
    pre-wash and pre-cut, 106
    as source of fiber, 52–54
vegetarian burger patties, 159, 181
vegetarian groups, 151
*Vegetarian Journal's Guide to Natural
    Restaurants in the* U. S. *and Canada*, 143
Vegetarian Nutrition Dietetic Practice
    Group, 146–147
Vegetarian Resource Group, 147
    web site for, 150

vitamin B12, 154
    sources of, 38
vitamin C
    sources of, 36
vitamin D, 154
    calcium and absorption of, 31–32
    supplements for, 38

W

water
    fiber and, 59
web sites
    about plant-based diets, 150
weight control
    consulting a registered dietitian, 49
    decreasing calorie intake, 43
    fat intake at 15–20% for, 68
    for kids, 50
    old view of, 41
    physical activity and, 42, 46
Wheat Foods Council, 7

Y

yogurt
    replacement for, 180